360 HEALTH

Your Guide to Cancer Prevention,
Healing Foods,
& Total Body Wellness

D1456758

by
Kimberly Maravich, RN

360 HEALTH

Your Guide to Cancer Prevention,
Healing Foods,
& Total Body Wellness

360 Health by Kimberly Maravich

Copyright © 2017 by Kimberly Maravich

Legal Disclaimer

To my adorable and loving sons, Nathan and Adam, who bring light, laughter, and love to my world. And to my husband Jim, who encourages and uplifts me every day.

In loving memory of my beautiful mother-in-law, Norma Jean, who lost her battle with cancer but leaves behind a legacy of joy and unconditional love.

"The tragedy of life is not death ...

but what we let die inside of us

while we live."

—Norman Cousins

Table of Contents

Introduction

Does cancer run in your family? Do you feel doomed to one day develop the disease? Are you unsure how to prevent major illnesses, or do you feel overwhelmed by the uncertainty of your future health? Is a friend or loved one dealing with a cancer scare or diagnosis? When it comes to cancer, there are seemingly endless questions. This book is designed to help you answer some of those questions and to give you well-researched insight into preventative health care.

The word "cancer" often elicits a visceral and gut-wrenching response. It is a term that invokes fear and panic in many people, largely because the cause is so uncertain, and sometimes, the prognosis is quite poor. On top of that, cancer can lie undetected in one's body for years, and a person may have no symptoms until the cancer has metastasized (spread) throughout the body. That is unnerving, to say the least.

You may be born with a particular set of genes, some that may factor into cancer development. However, those genes are not destined to manifest.

The study of "epigenetics" tells us that environmental factors (such as diet, lifestyle choices and behaviors, and stress) can change the health not only of the people who are exposed to them, but also the health of their descendants. The way you live can override bad genes! You can learn to "turn off" those genes with diet and lifestyle measures, measures which nourish your body and create an environment that makes it nearly impossible for cancer to grow. You need only to understand how to do that.

By adopting some of the prevention tactics provided in this book, you will begin to create your healthiest body, the body you were born to and deserve to inhabit.

Some of the ideas in this book are basic dietary changes that may or may not be difficult to follow, depending on your current diet. Some of the lifestyle changes that are suggested may challenge you to overhaul quite a few of your current practices, or they may reinforce what you're already doing. You may learn of beneficial supplements and herbs that you've never heard of before. You may learn that you need to avoid some of the household and beauty products you are currently using. You will learn about different ways to detoxify your body. There are also "alternative medicine" protocols listed to provide you with other views.

Some of the ideas may seem radical or even a little daunting. However, it is up to you to decide which suggestions to follow and which just are not your "cup of tea." A plethora of ideas will be provided so that you can be aware of what has worked for others to detoxify and ward off cancer. We'll also look at a large number of cancer research studies, rooted in science, that confirm for us the role of diet, supplements, and lifestyle in either predisposing us to cancer or helping us prevent cancer. At the end of each chapter, look for an "Anticancer Action" which is an easy first step you can take today to improve immunity and overall wellness.

Read the information and ideas and make a decision. Do you want to have the healthiest body possible? Do you want to lose weight and feel great in the process? Adopting even some of these suggestions will take you a long way in restoring your health and working to create a body in which cancer cannot thrive. It should go without mention that you should always consult your doctor to get his or her advice regarding any kind of dietary or lifestyle changes. Know that the information here is designed not to cure cancer but to benefit you by helping you to ward off disease and illness and to develop the body you were meant to have. Here's to your good health!

Chapter 1: How Cancer Forms

According to the National Cancer Institute, in 2016, it was estimated that a whopping 1,685,210 new cases of cancer would be diagnosed in the United States. Almost 600,000 people would die of the disease. The National Institutes of Health (NIH) also states that about 40% of the population will be affected by cancer at some point in their lives. Cancer mortality is higher among men than women; highest in African American males and lowest in Asian/Pacific Islander females.

The most common forms of cancer were projected to be breast cancer, lung and bronchus cancer, prostate cancer, colon and rectum cancer, bladder cancer, melanoma of the skin, non-Hodgkin lymphoma, thyroid cancer, kidney and renal pelvis cancer, leukemia, endometrial cancer, and pancreatic cancer. As you can see, cancer can affect just about any organ in the body.

These are staggering and scary statistics. However, the good news is there are risk factors which have been identified and linked with cancer growth. Knowing and avoiding the risk factors, and taking preventative measures will not only decrease your chances of developing the disease but will also allow you to experience overall good health.

What is Cancer?

By definition, cancer is a collection of diseases caused by an uncontrolled division of abnormal cells, resulting in malignant growths or tumors. Typically in the body, there is constant cell turn over; cells die and new ones are formed to replace them. However, when cancer develops, this normal process goes rogue. Older and damaged cells continue to thrive when they should die, and new cells form when they are not needed. These extra cells are abnormal and can divide without ceasing, turning into tumors or blood-born cancers. These tumors can also spread and be released into the body, metastasizing and invading other organs beyond the one of origin.

Depending on where the cancer is, different names are given. For example, there are carcinomas (the most common, made from cells that make up skin and the lining of internal organs), sarcomas (in bone and soft tissue), leukemias (in the blood-forming tissue of bone marrow), lymphomas (in white blood cells), myelomas (in plasma cells), melanomas (of the skin), and brain and spinal cord tumors to name a few. This book will not go into great detail about the various types of cancers because this is a book about prevention. However, it is important to note that regardless of the type, all cancers occur due to this abnormal cell division.

What Causes Abnormal Cells?

So what causes this creation and division of abnormal cells? To put it simply, normal cells and their DNA (genetic structure) are damaged. This damage can be an inherited genetic condition. However, according to the Mayo Clinic, most gene mutations occur after birth and are not inherited. Only a small percentage of cancers are actually passed down from the parents' genes. And even if you've acquired gene mutations, your lifestyle and exposures are what determine if the cancer will actually manifest. That means that cellular damage most likely is a result of environmental exposures to toxic materials, pollutants, infections, or foods.

This book will go into detail, covering most of the risk factors, why they are potentially dangerous, and how to best avoid them. The NIH lists the following risk factors for developing cancer:

* age
* alcohol consumption
* cancer causing substances
* chronic inflammation
* diet
* hormones

* immunosuppression
* infectious agents
* obesity
* radiation
* sunlight
* tobacco

These are among the risk factors this book will discuss. But we'll also look at other reasons cancer begins.

In general, the overarching cause for cancer is **inflammation**. There are many causative factors that contribute to inflammation, including the risk factors mentioned above. If you smoke, your body becomes inflamed. If you consume an acidic diet, full of refined and processed foods and oils, your body becomes inflamed. If you have chronic infections, your body becomes inflamed. If you are exposed to a lot of radiation and pollution, your body becomes inflamed. You get the idea.

Reducing total body inflammation is the goal in prevention of all cancers because over time, chronic inflammation can cause DNA damage that leads to cancer.

An article from *Nature: International Weekly Journal of Science*, published in 2002, analyzed a multitude of studies. The article states that inflammation is a critical component of tumor progression. It goes on to say that most cancers arise from infection, irritation, and inflammation. The article concludes by saying, "It is clear that anti-inflammatory therapy is efficacious towards early neoplastic progression and malignant conversion." In laymen's terms, this means that avoiding inflammation will help stop cancer from developing and/or spreading. The aim of this book is largely to teach you how to stop inflammation and start developing total body wellness.

What Causes Tumor Development and Metastasis?

Once abnormal cells are present, tumors can form. Have you heard of the term **angiogenesis**? Essentially, angiogenesis is the formation of new blood vessels. These new vessels begin in cancerous cells and can circulate blood to and from the rest of the body. This is quite dangerous because this is how metastasis works. The tumor now has a blood supply, rich with nutrients and energy to help it continue to thrive. And it can now spread to other organs.

Newer drugs are aimed at fighting angiogenesis. We will not discuss those medications in this book as they are aimed at treating pre-existing cancers. However, we will take a look at ways to stop angiogenesis dead in its tracks ... before cancer can even begin to thrive. We can create an internal environment that does not allow for tumor formation and growth. There are specific foods which are anti-angiogenic. By consuming a diet rich in these foods, we are ensuring that our bodies are fully capable of handling any assaults that may come its way. We can naturally boost our body's immune system and prevent blood vessels from forming that might feed microscopic tumors that exist.

Where Do We Begin the Fight Against Cancer and Move Toward Optimal Health?

We first need to look in depth at the risk factors involved in cancer formation. By knowing and addressing these, we can better prepare our bodies for optimal health and wellness. Then we can be proactive. We can add nourishing, non-acidic, anti-angiogenic foods to our diets. We can find ways to detox our bodies when needed. We can take supplements that are known to be anti-inflammatory and cancer-inhibitory. We can reduce stress and get rid of some of the outside stressors that attack us.

We can prepare our bodies to take on the world, remaining strong, disease-free, and feeling great.

---

* Anticancer Action *

Get a notebook, nothing fancy. As you read this book, write down five things from each chapter you find interesting and/or that you can begin to do tomorrow to improve your life and your health.

Chapter 2: Foods That Heal

Have you ever heard the adage, "Let food be thy medicine, and medicine be thy food?" This saying, dating back to 431 B.C., is attributed to Hippocrates, the father of medicine. In fact, today, doctors, upon graduation from medical school, take the Hippocratic Oath, affirming that they will treat their patients with dignity and as a whole person, not just a disease or condition. Albeit a part of antiquity, Hippocrates knew what mattered even then. Food can nourish and sustain, or it can cause illness and kill. Eating the right foods is THE MOST important thing we can do for our health.

It is common sense that some foods are much better for us than others. Our mothers always told us to "eat your vegetables," for good reason. Vegetables (and fruits, for that matter) are jam-packed with vitamins and minerals. Some are even anti-angiogenic, inhibiting cancer formation. We've also heard that eating fish is great for us. Healthy fats get bonus points as well. You could probably list a handful of foods that you already know to be beneficial. This chapter is dedicated to exploring the best of the best. Foods that not only nourish us and provide essential vitamins and minerals, but foods that also can help prevent a cancer diagnosis.

Anti-Angiogenic Foods

First, let's look at those foods that are known to inhibit angiogenesis (abnormal blood vessel formation that promotes and spreads cancerous tumors). These foods help to cut off the blood supply to tumors. Dr. William Li, an international expert in health and disease-fighting and the founder of the *Angiogenesis Foundation,* explains that certain foods can turn off the switch to cancer. "Tumor vessels, unlike healthy vessels, are abnormal and poorly constructed, and because of that, they're highly vulnerable to treatments that target them." He also says, "Mother Nature has laced a large number of foods, beverages and herbs with naturally occurring inhibitors of angiogenesis." Adding combinations of these foods to your diet will really help to create a healthy power-punch. Always try to buy them in their organic forms to avoid potential toxins. Below are lists of anti-angiogenic foods along with descriptions of some of their extra benefits.

1) Anti-Angiogenic Fruits

Red Grapes: The resveratrol in grapes has been shown to inhibit abnormal angiogenesis by 60%. Grapes contain powerful antioxidants known as polyphenols, which may slow or prevent many types of cancer.

Strawberries: The ellagic acid in strawberries is strongly anti-angiogenic. Strawberries are also full of antioxidants and other known cancer-fighters like folate and vitamin C.

Other Berries (Blueberries, Raspberries, and Blackberries): Berries' deep colors come from phytonutrients. These phytonutrients aid in the process of neutralizing free radical damage to our cells. They are also high in vitamins C and E.

Cherries: Cherries are high in quercetin and ellagic acid. This antioxidant flavonoid combo has been shown to promote cell and tissue health.

Citrus Fruits (Oranges, Lemons, Limes, and Grapefruit): Citrus fruits are filled with the flavonoids nobiletin and ascorbic acid (vitamin C). Both are anti-angiogenic.

Apples: The phytonutrients and antioxidants in apples help reduce the risk of developing cancer. Like many other fruits, apples are also high in fiber. Fiber is another cancer preventer.

Pineapple: A single serving of pineapple has more than 130% of the daily requirement of vitamin C for human beings, making it one of the richest and most delicious sources. Vitamin C is known for reducing illness and boosting the immune system.

Pumpkin: The beta-carotene in pumpkins, which gives it its orange hue, is a powerful immunostimulant. Beta-carotene can slow cancer growth, prevent DNA damage, and enhance enzymes which clear cancer-causing substances from the body.

2) Anti-Angiogenic Vegetables

Kale: Kale seems to have been "all the rage" for the past decade, and for good reason. It is loaded with vitamins and minerals. Most notably, it is a rich source of folate. Natural forms of folate are necessary for DNA synthesis and repair.

Bok Choy: There are over 70 antioxidants in this one food. Increased intake of antioxidants has been associated with decreased oxidative stress, thus lowering cancer risk.

Beets: Beets contain phytonutrients called betalains. Studies have shown that betalains help to protect the body from developing cancers such as lung, stomach, colon, and breast. Beets have anti-inflammatory properties and may also protect against heart disease. They are thought to assist in the body's detoxification process because they contain glutathione, a powerful antioxidant.

Artichokes: They are full of fiber and antioxidants. The phytonutrients in artichokes have also been found to interfere with estrogen receptor cancers. Rutin, quercetin, and gallic acid in artichokes are able to induce apoptosis, or cell death, within abnormal cells.

Parsley: This benign little garnish is actually a nutritional power house. It is rich in vitamins C, K, and A. It's also full of natural folate. Myricetin, a flavonoid in parsley, has been associated with skin cancer prevention. Another natural chemical, apigenin, has been shown to decrease tumor size.

Tomatoes: Fruit or vegetable? Whatever you call it, it's great for cancer prevention. Tomatoes are filled with lycopene, an antioxidant that is highly effective in scavenging cancer causing free radicals. Lycopene is better absorbed when tomatoes are heated and combined with healthy olive oil.

Garlic: Did you know Hippocrates himself prescribed garlic as medicine? It is a vegetable bulb, much like onions or leeks. It contains a compound called allicin which breaks down into sulfur. Sulfur is an important mineral because it helps our bodies detoxify and generate new, healthy tissues. It enables the transport of oxygen across cell membranes. Cancer hates oxygen. A sulfur deficiency also leads to inflammation, exactly what we are trying to avoid.

Maitake Mushrooms: Technically, mushrooms are not vegetables but a special type of fungus. Maitake mushrooms contain a polysaccharide fiber called beta glucan. The beta glucans work to activate and increase production of certain immune system cells such as macrophages, T-cells, natural killer cells, and neutrophils. These cells help to protect against illness and increase the body's resistance. Maitake mushrooms are also conveniently sold in powdered form. Health gurus suggest adding them to smoothies for an extra immune-system boost.

Soybeans: Again, soybeans are technically legumes and not vegetables. This one is controversial. Some doctors and nutritionists recommend staying away from soy products because of their estrogen-mimicking qualities. However, they have been found to be anti-angiogenic. Researchers believe that certain chemicals in soybeans called isoflavones are responsible for a lowered risk of breast cancer. Asian women, consuming high levels of soybeans, have a much lower incidence of breast cancer. The isoflavones are phytoestrogen (plant-based estrogen). However, it's been found that these actually "police" the estrogen in the body, inhibiting estrogen's effects if it is too high and supporting estrogen levels if they are too low. It is very important to buy organic soybeans. Soy is one of the most genetically modified (GMO) foods around.

3) Anti-Angiogenic Spices/Herbs

Turmeric: This is so important in cancer prevention that it's also sold in supplement/pill form. Turmeric gives curry its yellow color. Its main active ingredient is curcumin. Curcumin is a strong antioxidant which fights inflammation in the body. Multiple studies have shown that curcumin can kill a wide variety of tumor cells through diverse mechanisms.

Nutmeg: Nutmeg has been shown to induce cell death (apoptosis) in abnormal cells. This stops the spread of metastasis. Nutmeg also helps to detoxify the kidney and liver, increasing their overall function and making our bodies run more efficiently.

Lavender: Believe it or not, lavender can actually be eaten. (It is also an essential oil that we'll talk about in later chapters.) It can be used in baked goods, sauces, or salad dressings for added flavor. It is rich in vitamin A. It can also induce apoptosis, abnormal cell death, because it has a toxic effect on certain cancer cells.

Ginseng: Ginseng is a perennial herb. It contains ginsenosides which are its active anti-inflammatory components. Ginseng has been shown to repair DNA and inhibit cancer cell proliferation and tumors. It also improves T cells and NK cells (Natural Killer) in the human body which help with immunity.

Cinnamon: One of the most popular spices, cinnamon helps lower blood sugar.

It's also been found to interfere with tumors' blood supply.

Licorice: Now, we're not talking about RedVines candies here. We're referring to the extract from the actual sweet root plant. It is a great source of multiple vitamins and minerals. Studies have demonstrated that licorice roots restrict the growth of human cancers, specifically that of the breast.

4) Anti-Angiogenic Beverages

Green Tea: Green tea is loaded with antioxidants. Some powerful antioxidants are known as catechins. Green tea's major catechin is called EGCG. It is believed to be responsible for most of green tea's health benefits. In lab studies, EGCG was shown to be toxic to cancer cells and to actually prohibit them from growing. EGCG prevented the expression of a growth factor that is necessary for new blood-vessel development, thus shutting off the expansion of cancer cells.

Red Wine: Are you cheering now? Red wine is great for cancer prevention, in the right doses of course. Its polyphenols, catechins and resveratrol, are potent antioxidants. The polyphenols are found in the skins of grapes, which is why red wine is more beneficial. In the production of white wine, the skins are removed. Red wine's antioxidants protect against free radicals that have been implicated in the development of cancer.

5) Anti-Angiogenic Oils

Olive oil: You've probably heard that olive oil is one of the healthier oils to use. A study published in the journal *Molecular and Cellular Oncology* found that oleocanthal, the primary compound in extra virgin olive oil, eradicated cancer cells in less than an hour. Extra virgin olive oil is a good source of antioxidants and vitamins E and K that can protect the body from oxygen-free radicals and promote healthy cognitive function.

Grape Seed Oil: We've mentioned grapes and red wine made from grape skins, so it makes sense that the seeds might have benefits too. In lab studies on mice, researchers found that grape seed extract inhibited tumor growth in breast and other cancers. They also noted that it is well tolerated, so it may be used to develop medications that treat cancer.

6) Anti-Angiogenic Seafood

Tuna: You may have heard that tuna is rich in Omega-3s. You may have also heard that it is high in mercury. New research about mercury poisoning from tuna largely debunks that idea. Because tuna is also rich in selenium, it essentially counteracts mercury toxicity. Selenium binds with mercury, changing its composition so it isn't as dangerous. The high level of selenium is also what makes tuna cancer preventative. Selenium is a powerful antioxidant that works to neutralize free radicals before they can cause healthy cells to mutate.

Sea Cucumbers: Say what? Believe it or not, sea cucumbers are actually animals found on the ocean floor. They've been used in Chinese cuisine for centuries. They can be cooked and eaten, or dried and made into a powder. You can also buy sea cucumber capsules or liquid extract. Sea cucumbers have antibacterial and antiviral properties. They are also cytotoxic, meaning that they kill cancer cells.

7) Anti-Angiogenic Dessert

Dark Chocolate: Great news! Dark chocolate is packed with flavonoids, a group of phytochemicals that act as antioxidants. In fact, dark chocolate is one of the richest sources of antioxidants of any food. Be aware that milk chocolate is not the same, nor does it provide the same benefits. You'll need to consume 60-90% cacao to get the most bang for your buck. Extremely dark chocolate has higher amounts of antioxidants. You also want to avoid the sugars in milk chocolate. Dark and bittersweet chocolates are also much lower in sugars.

Other Super-Star Cancer-Inhibiting Foods

Next, we'll look at other foods which are also protective against cancer. Actually, depending on which resource you reference, some of the following foods may also be considered anti-angiogenic. Nevertheless, these foods may be equally effective in stopping cancer in its tracks because they are rich in antioxidants, vitamins, minerals, and essential micronutrients. Our body needs those to maintain stellar immunity.

1) Fruits

Honestly, you can't go wrong with pretty much any fruit. All fruits contain vitamins and nutrients that nourish our bodies. You may hear that you should be careful not to eat too many fruits in a day due to their high sugar content. But not all fruits are created alike and not all are high in sugars. If you can afford organic, that is the way to go for most fruits.

Fruits with thick skins like bananas, oranges, and avocados are less susceptible to pesticides, so you can buy the traditional versions.

Some fruits to consider adding to your diet are those rich in vitamin C. Vitamin C is a known immunity booster. Besides the citrus fruits and berries mentioned in the last section, the following fruits are also high in vitamin C, containing more than 20% of the Daily Value.

* **apricots, cantaloupe, guavas, kiwis, honeydew, papayas, watermelon**

Other known cancer-fighting, antioxidant-rich fruits are:

* **pomegranates, plums, prunes, raisins, cranberries**

Overall, adding more raw fruit to your diet will ensure that you're getting lots of vitamins, minerals, and antioxidants. All of these will help you create vibrant health.

2) Vegetables

Just like fruit, increasing the amount of vegetables in your diet will take you a long way toward good health. Vegetables are known for their cancer-fighting phytonutrients. Focus primarily on dark leafy greens which contain an abundance of folate and phytonutrients. Starchy vegetables may be equally as nourishing. Let's focus, for a moment, on different categories of vegetables and their benefits.

Dark, Leafy Greens: These are probably among the healthiest foods on the plant. Dark leafy green vegetables are bursting with carotenoids, folate, chlorophyll, and fiber. These compounds help stop or slow the growth of some forms of cancer. Chlorophyll is especially good at binding with carcinogens so that they can be eliminated by the body. It is important to try to buy greens in their organic forms. Due to their delicate leaves, they are quite susceptible to being contaminated by pesticides. They include, but are not limited to:

* **spinach, swiss chard, collard greens, turnip greens, mustard greens, rapini (broccoli rabe), romaine**

Cruciferous Vegetables: Some of the leafy greens listed above may overlap with this category on some lists. The word cruciferous means relating to the cabbage family. These veggies are also high in fiber, sulfur, and folate, and also in vitamins C, E, and K. Examples of these include:

* **kale, bok choy, watercress, broccoli, cabbage, arugula, brussels sprouts, cauliflower, radishes**

It is important to note that steaming broccoli and cauliflower actually releases more antioxidants. So they are better eaten cooked than raw.

Sulfur-Rich Vegetables: Sulfur is important because it's responsible for the body's ability to produce glutathione. Glutathione is an endogenous antioxidant, meaning that the body actually synthesizes it on its own. Glutathione is often referred to as "the master antioxidant" because it can regenerate itself in the liver and continue to attack free radicals. The cruciferous family also contains sulfur, but here we'll add on more. These are the allium family:

* onion, leeks, garlic, shallots

Sulfur is also important for the body's ability to detoxify. Eating these veggies actually helps you cleanse your system.

Orange Vegetables: Any foods that are orange by nature contain beta-carotene, a powerful antioxidant. (This applies to orange fruits, too.) Beta-carotene is a precursor to vitamin A. Vitamin A is a known immune system booster and helps to neutralize free radicals that attack the body. Orange foods also have vitamin C which, as previously mentioned, also supports the body's immunity.

* bell peppers, sweet potatoes, carrots, squash, pumpkin

3) Nuts

This category of food is beneficial to your health, as long as you have no allergies or food sensitivities to them. Nuts contain mono and polyunsaturated fats. They are also a source of Omega-3 fatty acids which are known to be heart healthy. They're filled with fiber and vitamin E. Some contain high levels of cancer-fighting antioxidants, too. Try to eat raw nuts when possible to avoid harmful and damaged oils. Dry roasted nuts are also fine and are typically just as healthy.

A 2015 Dutch study of 120,000 men and women ages 55-69 found that those who consumed a handful of nuts or peanuts (which are actually legumes) a day were less likely to die from diseases including cancer. Another 5-year study of 7,000 Spanish men and women ages 55-80 found that eating at least 3 servings of nuts per week reduced the risk of death from cancer.

Nut consumption appears to help prevent certain types of cancer. Breast, liver, colorectal, and pancreatic cancers have all been studied. Research shows that those who ate nuts are less susceptible to developing these cancers. Some nuts in particular also seem to be exceptionally beneficial.

Walnuts: One study cited in the journal *Nutrition Research and Practice* found that walnuts, eaten in conjunction with a Mediterranean-style diet (high consumption of vegetables and olive oil and moderate consumption of protein), greatly reduced inflammation and cancer. Walnuts contain ellagic acid which is a cancer-fighting antioxidant. Their phytosterols have been shown to block estrogen receptors in breast cancer cells. They appear to be protective against prostate cancer as well.

Pecans: Pecans are also extremely high in antioxidants. They contain vitamins and minerals like vitamins E and A, folate, calcium, magnesium, copper, phosphorus, potassium, manganese, B vitamins, and zinc. Their beneficial phytochemicals play an important role in removing toxic free radicals from the body. This helps to protect your body from disease and illness. Like walnuts, pecans also contain cancer-fighting ellagic acid.

Almonds: These nuts can cut cancer cell growth in half. This is largely studied in reference to breast cancer as found in a study published in *Gynecologic and Obstetric Investigation*. Almonds contain high levels of calcium and also magnesium, selenium, and vitamin E.

Peanuts: These are technically a legume but are often associated with nuts. (A legume is any plant that bears its fruit inside a pod.) There is some controversy when it comes to the mighty peanut. It is known to often contain a mold called aflatoxin which, as it sounds, is considered toxic. Some believe that toxin to be the cause of some allergies to peanuts. They are also often contaminated with pesticides. Therefore, it is best to buy organic peanuts and peanut butter (although peanut butter does not appear to have the same benefits as the nut). That being said, the same study cited above in *Gynecologic and Obstetric Investigation* found peanuts to be beneficial in helping to ward off breast cancer. And the 2015 Dutch study cited earlier also found a reduced death rate among those who frequently consumed peanuts.

Brazil Nuts: Due to their high selenium content, brazil nuts are helpful in warding off cancer and thyroid disease for that matter. A study outlined in the journal *Nutrition and Cancer* found that due to their high selenium levels, brazil nuts were, in fact, protective against cancer.

4) Seeds

Some seeds also appear to be beneficial in the fight against cancer.

Flaxseeds: Flax contains Omega-3s and lignans, powerful antioxidants. In petri dishes, lignans were found to have direct anticancer growth activity against breast cancer cells and against cell migration. A study conducted in 2005 also showed that flaxseed consumption reduced tumor growth in breast cancer patients.

Chia Seeds: Ch-ch-ch-chia! Remember that commercial? Chia seeds aren't just for growing crazy plants. They are entirely edible. Like flaxseeds, chia seeds also contain lignans. They've been studied and have been found to reduce the risk of hormone-dependent cancers like breast, prostate, uterine, and ovarian. Chia also contains ALA (alph-linolenic acid) which has been shown to induce apoptosis (cell death) in cancer.

Hemp Seeds: Although from the same family, hemp seeds are NOT the same as marijuana. So, feel free to unabashedly enjoy. Hemp seeds have been studied extensively. They've been found to help halt a deadly form of brain cancer, glioblastoma multiforme. Researchers also discovered they may help lung and breast cancer, too.

Sunflower Seeds: Studies show that the nutrients found in sunflower seeds have chemo-preventive compounds that stall early phases of cancer development to help shut off tumor growth. They are also a good source of vitamin E and selenium which help to ward off disease.

Apricot Seeds: Apricot seeds, also known as apricot kernels, contain amygdalin (vitamin B17). This vitamin is a powerful antioxidant. A concentrated form of amydalin is even used in the pharmaceutical Laetrile, which has been given in cancer clinics outside the United States.

Sprouts: Bean sprouts are just one type. Sprouted foods are known to be alkalizing. The vitamin C and chlorophyll contents are also increased when foods are sprouted.

5) Legumes

Legumes are sometimes controversial because of their effect on the digestive tract... think gas, bloating, indigestion. Those following a strict Paleo diet avoid legumes because they contain "anti-nutrients" like lectin and phytic acid. Lectins are thought to damage the lining of the small intestine and possibly also affect skeletal muscle. Phytic acid binds to minerals, so foods containing it do not lend to mineral absorption. Phytic acid also interferes with enzymes we need to digest our food. While they sound awful, they also have benefits. Phytic acid prevents the formation of free radicals, so it is an antioxidant. As for lectins, cooking beans and other legumes largely breaks them down, allowing them to be eaten without much issue. Soaking beans and cooking them can help to diminish some unwanted side effects. Also, limiting your intake of beans to 1-2 times a week and in small portions is enough to provide you with the benefits without all of the unpleasant side effects.

So what are the benefits of consuming legumes? The legumes listed below are among those in a category called "pulses." Pulses are actually seeds of legumes that use nitrogen from the atmosphere to make protein. Besides having protein and fiber, pulses also contain cancer fighting vitamins like folate. They contain phytochemicals and lignans (the powerful antioxidants mentioned in the section on seeds). Legumes are also considered to be resistant starches. This means they feed the good bacteria in the colon, creating an overall healthy digestive tract and protecting it from things like colon cancer.

   * **Kidney and black beans, split peas, and lentils**

6) Resistant Starches

Let's look a little deeper at resistant starches. What are they exactly? By definition, resistant starches are carbohydrates that resist digestion in the small intestine and enter into the large intestine, or colon, mostly in the same form they entered your mouth. They can ferment in the colon to promote the growth of "good" bacteria. By various mechanisms, they might also assist in the prevention of cancers. Basically, these starches ferment in the gut, creating a lower pH. Not only does this allow good bacteria to proliferate, but it also wards off harmful, pathogenic bacteria. Essentially, resistant starches act as probiotics. They have been found to be helpful in fighting off colon cancer and even breast cancer. There are different types of resistant starches, but all have about the same function in our bodies. In addition to legumes, the following foods are also considered resistant starches:

   * **green bananas, plantains, al dente whole grain pasta, pumpernickel bread, rolled oats, cereals like muesli, peas, cooked and cooled potatoes, rice, sweet potatoes, potato starch, tapioca**

7) Fermented Foods

Resistant starches act like probiotics and so do fermented foods. In fact, fermented foods ARE probiotics. They contain a host of beneficial bacteria. Probiotics are absolutely necessary for sustaining gut health. Good gut flora helps to ensure a robust immune system. A Finnish study found that the fermentation process involved in making sauerkraut, for example, produces several cancer-fighting compounds. One of the ways cancer develops is through exposure to carcinogens, some of which can be ingested or generated by an abundance of harmful gut flora. Probiotic foods can help remove the exposure to those carcinogens by detoxifying the body, inhibiting tumor growth, and stimulating the immune system.

* sauerkraut, pickles, kimchi, kombucha, yogurt and kefir (made from dairy or coconut), tempeh, miso

8) Spices/Herbs

There are a number of spices that can contribute to your daily antioxidant dose. Each has its own perk. The beauty of cooking with spices is that they're often combined, giving the food greater health benefits as well as adding extra flavor.

In the above section on anti-angiogenic foods, we already mentioned the benefits of **turmeric, nutmeg, lavender, cinnamon, and licorice**. These spices are known to inhibit cancer growth and blood flow to tumors.

The book *Herbal Medicine: Biomolecular and Clinical Aspects* by Iris Benzie and Sissi Wachtel-Galor discusses dozens of spices used in the treatment and prevention of cancer. Let's look at a few of these in regard to their association with the immune system.

Allspice: Allspice possesses antimicrobial, antioxidant, analgesic, and anticancer properties. Allspice reduces inflammation, thus reducing the risk of cancer. It contains a multitude of potential bioactive agents that may contribute to health promotion, including flavonoids, phenolic acids, and catechins.

Allspice has a warm, peppery flavor. You can use allspice in chai tea; in sweet dishes that need a little spiciness, like gingerbread; or to make jerk chicken.

Basil: Basil is a potent antimicrobial. In fact, it's been used in the treatment of H. pylori, a bacterial stomach infection. It's been shown to both lower oxidative damage and decrease skin tumors in mice.

Among its many uses, basil is often mixed with pine nuts, olive oil, and parmesan cheese to make pesto.

Caraway: Caraway is a proven antioxidant. Animal models have been used to explore the anticancer potential of caraway in cancers of the colon and skin. Caraway has antifungal properties and is sometimes used to treat candida.

Caraway is the seed often used in rye bread and certain forms of sauerkraut. It has a flavor profile similar to licorice.

Cardamom: A member of the ginger family, cardamom is a known antioxidant. In a study with Swiss albino mice, it decreased liver tumors. It's also been shown to decrease colon carcinogens by its anti-inflammatory and proapoptotic (cancer cell death) activities.

My mother always used cardamom in a delicious Finnish braided bread. It is also a common ingredient in Indian foods. It can be combined with other spices to make sweet or savory dishes. It is spicy and citrusy, and goes well with cinnamon, nutmeg, or allspice.

Clove: In mice studies, clove was found to help with cellular detox in the liver, stomach, and esophagus. Evidence also suggests that clove may help prevent colon cancer. It contains eugenol, a potent anti-inflammatory.

Whole cloves are often placed in ham while it cooks for added flavor. You can also purchase ground cloves. They are used for seasoning meats, stews, and sauces; for desserts with berries like pies or fruitcakes; and in warm beverages like teas or cider.

Coriander/Cilantro: Coriander seeds are known to help the hepatic system (liver) detoxify. It's also been used for skin inflammation and can help ward off colon cancer. Depending on the part of the world in which you live, coriander is also known as cilantro. Cilantro can help detoxify heavy metals from the body. It contains quercetin, which is a known anti-inflammatory, and protects against free radical damage.

Cilantro is a leafy herb. It is often used in Mexican dishes like guacamole. It has a very fresh flavor, so it's great in salads. It also has a cooling feel and is sometimes added as a garnish to spicier dishes.

Coriander seeds, on the other hand, are a different part of the plant and are much more sour. They are often used in pickling, spices, and herb blends.

Cumin: Cumin has been reported to exhibit antioxidant, antimicrobial, anti-inflammatory, and chemo-preventive properties (delaying or inhibiting the development of cancer). In lab studies, it's been shown to ameliorate cancer in the stomach. Evidence also suggests that cumin may suppress tumor cells, including colorectal, breast, bone, ovarian, pancreatic, and myeloblastic leukemia.

Cumin is a major component of curries and taco seasonings. It's used in making falafel and Indian dishes, too.

Dill: Like other spices, dill is used for detoxification purposes. Dill has been shown to reduce DNA damage and inhibit estrogen metabolism in laboratory studies. Dill also protects against free radicals.

Dill often accompanies and seasons fish. It's also used as a garnish or added to salad dressings or dips. It goes well with potato salad. And, of course, it's used in making dill pickles.

Ginger: Worldwide, ginger is consumed not only as a spice but also as medicine. Several studies have investigated ginger's antioxidant properties. In lab studies, rats stricken with cancer were administered ginger. After 26 weeks, the rats given ginger had significantly less cancerous tumors. In a study out of Georgia State, mice given ginger extract had a 56% reduction in prostate tumor size.

Fresh ginger is used commonly in stir fries, sauces, marinades, and Indian curries. It's used in hot teas and ginger beers or ales. It's also great for baked goods like gingerbread, cakes, or pies.

Rosemary: The journal *Critical Reviews in Food Science and Nutrition* lists a review of studies from 1996 to 2010. The studies found that rosemary had an ability to suppress the development of tumors in several organs including the colon, breast, liver, and stomach, as well as melanoma and leukemia cells.

Rosemary is an herb often roasted with meats and potato dishes. It can also be used in focaccia bread, tomato sauces, and with olive oil to enhance foods' flavor.

Saffron: Scientists are finding that saffron has the unique ability to both slow and reverse cancer growth. A growing body of literature now supports the use of saffron for the prevention of several of the most aggressive and deadly human cancers, including liver, lung, and stomach cancers.

Saffron is especially good in cooking seafood dishes such as bouillabaisse and paella. It is also used in risotto and other rice dishes.

Thyme: Thyme has been studied for its effects on liver carcinoma cells and colon cancer cells. Thyme possesses terpenoids which are recognized for their cancer preventive properties.

Thyme is used as a seasoning for meat, particularly poultry and pork. It can also be used in potato and rice dishes. It's often used in Italian, French, and Mediterranean cooking.

Protein Sources

You may have heard it said that following a vegetarian or vegan diet is helpful in preventing cancer. Undoubtedly, research supports following a heavily produce-based diet, rich in fruits and vegetables, which nourish our bodies with antioxidants and micronutrients that prevent cancer. However, there are certain sources of protein that appear to be protective against the disease. Also, when protein is combined with other foods at meals, it works to stabilize blood sugar. Remember that cancer feeds off of sugars. By reducing overall carbohydrate loads (especially carbs from refined foods) and adding more quality fats and moderate amounts of protein, our bodies will have better blood sugars and a more robust immune system.

One caveat is that the animal protein we consume should be the purest, cleanest forms we can find. What does that mean? We need to look for fish that are wild caught and not farm raised. Our beef products, when possible, should be organic and grass-fed. Likewise, chicken and eggs should be organic and pasture-raised. Other meats like pork and lamb are also best bought in their natural forms, without antibiotics or hormones. In the next chapter, we'll explore the reasons why we need to avoid certain fish and meats and why antibiotics, hormones, and conventional animal-feeds are harmful.

9) Seafood

In the section on anti-angiogenic foods, we listed tuna and sea cucumbers as seafood that actually stops blood vessel formation to potential cancer cells. Other members of the fish and seafood family offer benefits that can be protective from cancer.

Oily Fish: Remember to look for the wild caught varieties of these fish as they are purer and cleaner. Oily fish tend to be higher in Omega-3s. Omega-3s are powerful anti-inflammatories in the body that minimize COX-2, an enzyme responsible for inflammation and for driving cancer and metastases. Omega-3s have been shown to re-lengthen DNA telomeres, which shorten when you have cancer.

Salmon also has an antioxidant called astaxanthin. It is ten to twenty times more powerful than many other carotenoids. Astaxanthin is responsible for giving salmon its reddish hue. In an article in the journal *Marine Drugs*, researchers found that astaxanthin shows clinical promise in anti-tumor therapy and may be preventative to various types of cancer.

* salmon, herring, trout, mackerel, sardines

10) Meat

Meat is a relatively touchy subject when it comes to cancer prevention. There is an entire group of thinkers who believe that no meat is better than some. The belief is that meat consumption predisposes one to cancer because it is devoid of fiber, and it can release carcinogenic compounds when cooked at high temperatures. Harvard studies showed that daily meat eaters have approximately three times the colon cancer risk, compared to those who rarely eat meat. It's also been shown that in countries consuming a diet higher in saturated fat and meat, women tend to have higher rates of breast cancer. In the next chapter, we'll look closer at types and preparations of meat that may be considered dangerous or may contribute to cancer.

Some of these studies, however, are observational in nature and do not consider the entire diet of those studied. For example, did those studied eat diets also high in sugar? Did they also eat processed foods? Chris Kresser, leader in nutrition and author of the book *Your Personal Paleo Code,* explains that a person's overall gut micro biome is more important for sustaining health and that modest protein consumption is not only fine but is advisable for health benefits. In his blog post "Red Meat & Cancer - Again! Will It Ever Stop?", he largely debunks the thought that meat causes cancer. Meat contains a myriad of vitamins, amino acids, and minerals. It can be a part of a nourishing diet, just as our ancestors followed.

So, the question remains, are any meats actually considered to be cancer protective?

Lamb: Lamb is actually considered to one of the cleanest sources of meat. It contains vitamins B12, B3, selenium, zinc, iron, and phosphorous. Believe it or not, lamb is also a good source of Omega-3s. It contains conjugated linoleum acid (CLA) which is responsible for reducing inflammation and boosting the immune system.

Grass-Fed Beef: This type of beef is preferable because the cattle are consuming what nature intended them to eat. Their digestive tracts are designed to eat grass. Grass-fed cows are less sick and do not require antibiotics. They are typically raised on farms that do not use pesticides. They are not given hormones. Grass-fed beef contains three to five times the amount of CLA as conventional, grain-fed beef. They, too, are a source of Omega-3s. Look for grass-finished beef as well. This means that the cows are permitted to graze and eat grass throughout their entire life span, and they are overall much healthier than grain-fed or grain-finished animals.

Organ Meats: Do you eat liver? How about heart or kidney? Did you know our ancestors ate animals "nose to tail"? This means that all parts of the animals were consumed, including organs. In fact, muscle meats (like the beef, chicken, and pork we know) were given to dogs or discarded at times because they weren't as desirable. Seems our ancestors knew that organ meats provided many essential nutrients, above and beyond muscle meats. Organic liver, for example, is rich in vitamins E, A, B12, D, selenium, zinc, folate, iron, and Omega-3s.

Notice a trend in referencing the importance of Omega-3 fats? As mentioned earlier, Omega-3s help with DNA formation. They are "essential" fatty acids because our bodies cannot produce them, but we need them. Omega-3s help our cells maintain their structure, and they help reduce inflammation. And remember, inflammation leads to cancer.

Make sure that you are consuming only organ meats from organically raised animals and from grass-fed cattle. Our livers work to detoxify our bodies; so do animals' livers. We want to ensure we are eating the cleanest and healthiest organ meats around so they can nourish our bodies, not deliver unwanted toxins.

Bone Broth: Bone broth is made from the bones of (preferably) grass-fed cattle or bison or pastured chicken. The bones are simmered in filtered water for long periods of time, think 12-24 hours or more. Also added to the water is perhaps some salt and vegetables like carrots and onions for flavor, and a bit of apple cider vinegar. The vinegar is very important because it allows the simmering bones to leech minerals into the broth. These minerals are precisely why bone broth is so nutritive and is often referred to as "nature's multi-vitamin."

Bone broth is one of the most nourishing foods on the planet. Have you ever heard the adage, "Eat what ails you"? Well, by consuming bone broth, we get all of the benefits of the animal's bones and connective tissues. Bone broth helps strengthen our hair, nails, and bones. The gelatin found in bone broth also heals our digestive tracts. Best of all, it boosts our immunity and decreases inflammation. There is a reason why our mothers and grandmothers gave us homemade chicken soup when we were sick. Bone broth has those same wonderful minerals that restore our health. Amino acids (glycine, proline, and arginine) in the broth have anti-inflammatory effects.

11) Dairy Products

As you'll see, not all dairy is created equal. Some dairy products are cancer fighters. Others, depending on how they are sourced and how the dairy cows were raised, are potentially toxic.

Whey Protein: When we consider whey, it is important to note that we are not referring to the sugar-laden or artificially sweetened post-workout powders and bars. Look for a high-quality, pasture-raised, organic, cold-processed, non-denatured whey protein concentrate ... free of GMO ingredients like soy, corn, and wheat as well as chemicals, artificial colors, and sweeteners.

Whey contains lactoferrin which is a cancer killer and activates the innate immune system cells like the neutrophils, macrophages, and T-cells. These are the first line of defense against harmful pathogens, including cancer cells. Lactoferrin also triggers the production of glutathione, better known as the "master" antioxidant and a powerful substance in the prevention of cancer.

Yogurt: As for yogurt, scientists have found that the active culture of bacteria in yogurt, Lactobacillus, actually helps to fortify the immune system. Studies have shown that the use of yogurt in the diet triples the internal production of interferon which the immune system uses against tumor cells. Yogurt has also been shown to raise the level of natural killer cells and to slow down the growth of tumor cells in the GI tract. Choose brands that state "contains live and active cultures" on the package. Avoid sweetened yogurt due to the high sugar content. Also go for organic yogurt, and if possible, from grass-fed cows.

Kefir: Kefir is a fermented milk drink made from kefir "grains." The grains are a gelatinous mass harboring a generous variety of bacteria and yeast from which one can make continual batches of kefir. Kefir is an even more potent source of probiotics than yogurt as it has over 30 strains of bacteria. It has a slightly sour taste. Because it is sour, manufacturers may add a significant amount of sugar. Be careful not to buy kefir that contains too much sugar, as this will potentially counteract its benefits.

In a 2007 study out of China, researchers found anti-proliferative effects of kefir on human breast cancer cells. After six days of exposure, the cancer cells stopped spreading. Also a 2015 review of 11 studies on kefir found that kefir consistently showed beneficial effects on cancer prevention and treatment. These cancers included breast, colon, skin, stomach, and leukemia and, in experimental studies, on different sarcomas.

12) Eggs

Eggs are a food that YOU will need to decide whether or not to eat. That may be confusing, but science is not consistent with this. Eggs are often considered allergenic. Many people have histamine reactions to them, but others have subtler sensitivities to them. If you react in any way, you must avoid them. Below, we will list some of the benefits of eggs, but you'll also find in the next chapter that eggs will also be referenced as potential foods to avoid. Read all the information and references to studies and make an informed decision.

To start, don't worry about the cholesterol in eggs. Studies show that the cholesterol we ingest from animal products does not contribute to our inherent cholesterol levels. Cleveland Clinic cardiologist Dr. Steven Nissen estimates that only 20% of your blood cholesterol levels come from your diet. The rest of the cholesterol in your body is produced by your liver. Sugar and carbohydrate intake play a much greater role. There is a direct correlation between insulin and cholesterol levels. So following a lower carbohydrate diet would benefit one more if he or she were trying to reduce cholesterol. However, you should also be aware that your body *needs* cholesterol. Our cell membranes, our nerve encasings, and our brains are all made up of cholesterol.

The yolks of eggs are the important part when it comes to cancer prevention. Researchers from the University of Alberta determined that egg yolks in their raw state contain almost twice as many antioxidant properties as an apple. When fried or boiled, however, antioxidant properties were reduced by about half. Hmm ... who eats raw eggs?

Let's look a bit further. Eggs contain choline. Choline is an essential micronutrient. Studies consistently find that people with diets rich in choline have the lowest levels of inflammatory markers such as IL-6, TNF-alpha, and C-reactive protein. Additionally, people that eat a choline-deficient diet for as short as a month have been found to have a significant increase in DNA damage and cancer risk.

Choline seems to be especially beneficial for prevention of breast cancer. A study from the University of North Carolina of more than 3,000 adult women found a 24% reduced risk of developing breast cancer in women with the highest intake of choline compared to women with the lowest intake. Another study from 2005 found a 44% lower risk for developing breast cancer in women who ate at least six eggs per week when compared to women who ate two or less eggs per week.

So, if breast cancer runs in your family, you may want to introduce more eggs into your diet. Remember, consuming eggs from organic, pastured chickens is the preferred choice. This ensures the eggs are not given antibiotics or toxic feeds. Eggs from pastured hens also have twice as much vitamin E and long-chain omega-3 fats, and vitamin A concentration is also about 38% higher.

13) Beverages

There are some drinks worth mentioning when it comes to cancer protection. These may be often overlooked but are just as important in one's diet and overall health.

Juices/Smoothies: Juicing is considered one of the easiest and most effective ways to get fresh, raw, organic fruits and vegetables into our systems. Please note that we are not speaking of most store-bought juices as they are typically filled with sugars or artificial sweeteners, artificial colors, synthetic ingredients, and possibly GMOs. With a few rare store-bought exceptions (most likely in the refrigerated section of the produce aisle), we are primarily referring to the juices you blend and create at home.

Almost all of the benefits of fruits and vegetables are extended into their juices; all of the vitamins and minerals that are so crucial in cancer prevention. If one already has cancer, juicing is recommended as a way to get nourishment without having to do much digestion while giving the body quick energy. Juicers remove the pulp of the produce and just expel the liquid in a very concentrated form.

However, if you're looking for ways to prevent cancer and other illness, using the fruits and vegetables to create smoothies is probably the way to go. Smoothies simply blend the fruits and veggies with something like water, coconut water, almond milk, or coconut milk and are consumed with all of the fiber. The fiber helps to slow any spike in blood sugar, and it also provides roughage to help detoxify and cleanse the colon and digestive tract. As with juices, buying store-bought smoothies may also be dangerous due to added sugars and sweeteners, so it's best to make these at home.

Coffee: Studies show that coffee can reduce the risk of developing several cancers: endometrial, liver, colorectal, and melanoma. One study found that drinking three to four cups of coffee a day could reduce the risk of endometrial cancer by almost a fifth. In another study out of Italy, researchers found that coffee consumption can decrease the occurrence of liver cancer by 40%. It is also widely understood that coffee decreases the risk of developing cirrhosis of the liver. One study of 489,706 individuals found that those who drank more than four cups of coffee per day had a lower risk of colorectal cancer. In a 2014 study of over 400,000 Caucasians, researchers found that those who consumed more than four cups of coffee per day had a 20% reduction in the risk of melanoma compared to those who consumed no coffee.

Coffee is known for its abundance of antioxidants. According to an article cited in the *Journal of Nutrition*, the single greatest dietary contributor to total antioxidant intake is coffee, above and beyond consumption of fruits and vegetables. Antioxidants are important because they help prevent cell damage and inflammation and lower the risk of developing certain diseases.

Black Tea: We've seen that green tea is anti-angiogenic, but black tea also has anticancer properties. In a 2015 study, researchers found that a natural extract from black tea (BTE) possessed anti-proliferative qualities against colon cancer and breast cancer. Black tea contains polyphenols, which are antioxidants that help block DNA damage. It also contains alkylamine antigens that help boost our immune response.

Dandelion Tea: This is an herbal tea with a surprisingly mellow flavor. Dandelion tea has been used as a medicinal herb for centuries across many different cultures. It contains vitamins A, C, and D, as well as zinc, iron, magnesium, and potassium. It also has bioactive compounds with potential anticancer properties. In isolated studies, it was shown to ward off pancreatic cancer, melanoma, and certain forms of leukemia.

Alcohol: Now, don't get overly excited about this one. Yes, we did see earlier that red wine is, in fact, anti-angiogenic. And other forms of alcohol may also benefit us in other ways. However, alcohol must be consumed in the right amounts for it to be therapeutic.

Alcohol can protect against the bacteria Helicobacter pylori which is known to cause ulcers and may lead to stomach cancer. A study from Queens University found that drinking three to six glasses of wine or one to two half-pints of beer a week showed 11% fewer infections of H. pylori.

Consuming too much alcohol, however, is associated with increased risks of mouth, throat, esophageal, liver, and breast cancers. A common recommendation is to consume no more than one to two drinks per day. However, most researchers agree that one to two drinks *per week* is preferable when it comes to cancer prevention. If you have a history of alcoholism or excessive binge-drinking tendencies, you are probably better off avoiding alcohol all together due to its potentially addictive properties.

Pure Filtered Water: In the next chapter we'll look in depth at why unfiltered water can be downright dangerous to our health. However, for now, it's important to note that pure filtered water, and lots of it, is helpful in our fight against cancer. For one, water helps us to detoxify our bodies. It promotes healthy digestion and flushes our colons, eliminating toxins. Water also provides nourishment for the body's cellular system. Without water, our cells cannot do their jobs and remain healthy. Research published in the *Journal of Clinical Oncology* reveals that water intake is inversely related to bladder, colon, and breast cancers; meaning the more water a person drinks, the less likely he or she is to develop these potentially fatal conditions.

Lemon Water with Himalayan Sea Salt: Are you telling us to salt our lemon water? Yes! There are anticancer benefits to both lemons and Himalayan sea salt that, when combined, create a powerhouse duo. Lemons are rich in the antioxidant vitamin C, and phagocytes and T-cells rely on vitamin C to perform their tasks of protecting the body and helping with immunity. Himalayan sea salt is rich in nourishing trace minerals; 84 to be exact. Regular table salt is devoid of these minerals. Dr. Linus Pauling, a two-time Nobel Prize winner said, "You can trace every sickness, every disease, and every ailment to a mineral deficiency." When you add lemon juice to the salted water, the vitamin C helps the body to more efficiently absorb specific nutrients, making them more bioavailable. So, combining the lemon water with sea salt helps the body take in all of the health sustaining minerals it needs.

Again, you need to begin with pure filtered water. Take a pinch of granulated Himalayan sea salt, and stir it into the water. Then add the juice of half a lemon. I like to warm my water in a mug before adding the salt and lemon, and I drink it first thing in the morning. This ensures that I'm getting all the goodness on an empty stomach, and it often helps to get the day "moving" along. You can also make a brine of "Sole" water (pronounced *so-lay*) to keep and add this to your water and lemon juice each day. Sole water is just water, kept at room temperature in a plastic-lid mason jar that is oversaturated with Himalayan sea salt crystals such that the crystals remain at the bottom and do not dissolve. Each day, add a teaspoon of the brine to your water, then add lemon. The Sole brine is shelf-stable and does not require refrigeration because the salt makes it antibacterial in nature.

Apple Cider Vinegar: Of course, you won't actually drink apple cider vinegar straight up by itself. That would burn your esophagus. But apple cider vinegar (ACV) diluted in water has benefits. Some lab studies on rats have shown ACV's potential for killing cancer cells. ACV is known to be antibacterial, antiviral, and antifungal. Raw, organic, unfiltered ACV with the "mother" (the starter) is thought to be best since it's in the most unadulterated, purest form. Among its many benefits, ACV can alkalinize the body, regulate blood sugar, improve heart health by lowering blood pressure and raising HDL, provide antioxidants, help detoxify the liver, ease digestion, accelerate weight loss, and decrease osteoporosis risk by improving calcium absorption.

14) Fats

Believe it or not, certain fats are exceptionally desirable for our body's functioning. Our cell membranes are composed of fats, so having healthy cells is dependent on having healthy dietary fats.

Olive Oil: Olive oil can help to reduce damage to your genes and protect against cancer. A study in the scientific journal *Molecular & Cellular Oncology* found an antioxidant compound in olive oil, called oleocanthal, kills cancer cells rapidly, in as little as thirty minutes in the laboratory. Extra Virgin olive oil contains the greatest concentration of naturally-occurring antioxidants.

Coconut Oil: Coconut oil contains lauric acid which is a medium-chain fatty acid that supports the immune system and has antimicrobial properties. A study published in the journal *Cancer Research* showed that the lauric acid in coconut oil completely exterminated more than 90% of colon cancer cells after just two days of treatment in vitro (in petri dishes).

Avocado: Avocados are an excellent source of healthy monounsaturated fat, vitamins, and antioxidants. In a recent study published in the journal *Cancer Research*, a type of fat found in avocados was found to combat acute myeloid leukemia (AML). The California Avocado Commission states that avocados contain 11 carotenoids. They say, "Carotenoids appear to protect against certain cancers, heart disease, and age-related macular degeneration." Another study, out of Ohio State University, found that avocados can also ward off oral cancer by killing oral cancer cells while leaving normal cells alone. Essentially avocados signal cancer cells to self-destruct (apoptosis).

Final Thoughts on Healing Foods to Eat and Enjoy

We've just explored an exhaustive catalog of foods with proven benefits against cancer. If you're feeling overwhelmed, please don't. Of course, you couldn't possibly incorporate each and every food on these lists into your diet. And you probably wouldn't want to. You may not care for liver, mushrooms, broccoli, etc. That's okay! Pick as many foods as you like and feel comfortable including in your diet. Perhaps you first increase the overall amount of fruits and veggies you are eating. Then try adding in some varieties you've never eaten before. Maybe you could integrate more spices into your cooking. You could try starting your day with a fortifying smoothie, filled with fruit, veggies, avocado, and flax. Try a snack of nuts and green tea. Add coconut oil to your coffee. Start where you are and with the diet you're accustomed to, and slowly make little changes toward better nutrition. You may just be surprised how well you can feel!

One last note, you may be concerned about the cost of buying organic and grass-fed products. In the next chapter, we'll get to the importance of why grass-fed, antibiotic-free, and hormone-free meats are better options and much, much healthier not only for the animals but for you. As far as fruits and vegetables are concerned, you've probably heard of the "dirty dozen." These are the 12 most commonly contaminated fruits and veggies. At the bare minimum, be sure that the following foods are almost always consumed in their organic states: **apples, celery, bell peppers, peaches, strawberries, nectarines, grapes, spinach, lettuce, cucumbers, blueberries, and potatoes**. Fruits and veggies not on this list may be bought in their conventional forms if you're eating on a budget.

When you cut back on refined, packaged, and sugary foods to opt for products "closer to nature" like meats, fish, fruits, and vegetables, you will also cut back on part of your grocery bill. Think of it this way, you are making an investment in your health and in the health of your family when you buy the best quality and most nourishing foods available. Healthcare (or "sick care") costs for the management of existing diseases can bankrupt a family. Where would you rather spend your money?

---

* Anticancer Action *

The next time you are at the grocery store, buy one fruit and one vegetable you've never tried before.

Over the course of each week, try to eat the "rainbow." Choose red, orange, yellow, green, blue, and purple produce.

Chapter 3: Foods to Limit or Avoid

The last chapter had us feeling excited about incorporating some new, wonderfully healthy foods into our meal plans. But, we'd be remiss if we didn't devote time to focusing on what to remove from our diets. Whereas as some foods can heal us, others can sicken us. Unfortunately, some of those illness-causing foods are delicious, addictive, and frequently consumed.

One of the biggest favors you can do for yourself on your path towards health and vitality is to get rid of "garbage" foods. If you sometimes (or often) eat junk foods, you're not alone. Our society turns a blind eye to the junk we put into our bodies. We've become numb to it all, and sometimes we don't even think about what we're eating. But, it's not entirely our fault! Our stores are stocked with every processed, refined, hydrogenated, salt and sugar-laden substance you could ever imagine. The Standard American Diet is just that ... SAD! And sadly, you cannot be healthy when you're eating an unhealthy diet. "You are what you eat." This is the truth! Every cell, every muscle, every organ is partially composed of what enters our mouths and what "nourishes" us.

When you understand **why** the foods listed in this chapter are not the healthiest options, it will help you make better decisions. We may have heard a particular food is "bad" for us, but we often don't know why. This chapter is an effort to help shine a spotlight on potentially toxic foods ...

so you can be a smarter consumer. And so you can create your healthiest body.

Keep an open mind while reading through the list of these foods. Know that you wouldn't be expected to avoid every single one, but limiting your exposure or reducing the amount of these you eat will do you well. Your body will thank you!

1) Some Meat Products

Of course, not all kinds of meat are bad for you. We listed some very nourishing meats and fish in the last chapter such as grass-fed beef and salmon. But other types may not be fine. Some of the problems are in the preparation of these meat products, the way they are cooked or preserved. Some problems are due to the way the animals were raised and what they were fed. Other issues, according to some researchers, lie in the inherent nature of what meat is and its macronutrient content. We'll explore all of these ideas.

Charbroiled and Grilled: Cooking meat at very high temperatures, especially to the point of blackening, changes its molecular structure. It causes harmful chemicals like HCAs (heterocyclic amines) and PAHs (polycyclic aromatic hydrocarbons) to form. These chemicals are carcinogenic, meaning that they are capable of changing DNA structure to create cancerous cells. (Note that this does NOT apply to grilled vegetables. They do not develop carcinogens.) In many experiments, rodents fed a diet supplemented with HCAs developed tumors of the breast, colon, liver, skin, lung, prostate, and other organs. Rodents fed PAHs also developed cancers, including leukemia and tumors of the gastrointestinal tract and lungs. During this research, the rodents were fed large amounts of these carcinogens.

The take away message is to limit your exposure to meat cooked at very high temperatures. That will ensure you're not getting an abundance of carcinogens. Instead, try eating more baked, boiled, slow-roasted, and slow-cooked meat. Crock-Pots are wonderful for this!

If you must grill, be sure to cut away the charred parts. Keep flipping meats continuously to ensure quick and even cooking. Cut back on how often you grill; maybe only do so a few times a month. Another tip is to marinate your meat before grilling. You do NOT want to use pre-made marinades that contain a lot of sugar. Adding sugar to the meat before grilling actually *triples* the amount of HCAs. Instead, create your own marinades using spices and herbs (some of which might just be anti-carcinogenic), and use a vinegar-based sauce. Rosemary has been shown to greatly reduce these harmful chemicals. You could also soak your meat in wine prior to grilling.

Pickled, Smoked, and Processed: These types of preparations also damage the structure of meat. There is an association between gastric cancer and pickled products. According to the journal *Cancer Epidemiology, Biomarkers & Prevention*, consuming pickled foods results in a 50% increased risk of stomach cancer. Those studied were mainly from Eastern Asia (China, Japan, Korea) who often consume pickled meats and vegetables.

The harmful component of most processed meat is the nitrate content. These are preservatives that help to prolong shelf life. However, the additives used in these processed foods can accumulate in your body over time and cause damage at the cellular level, leading to cancer. Cured meat, which consists of jerky, bacon, sausage, salami, corned beef, and ham all contain chemicals that help with processing. There is an association between these and bowel cancer.

Smoking meats has basically the same effect as grilling meats at high temperatures. Researchers studied a population in Hungary over 10 years. This population consumes a high amount of home-smoked meats. The incidence of stomach cancer was 50% higher than the average population of those not consuming smoked meat.

In 2015, the World Health Organization (WHO) came out with recommendations regarding processed meat. These were based on the International Agency for Research on Cancer (IARC) findings that reviewed over 800 studies of people who daily consumed processed meat. Researchers found a direct correlation between colorectal cancer and consumption of such meat. The equivalent consumption causing cancer was four strips of bacon or one hot dog per day. However, the WHO did not recommend completely eliminating these meats. Professor Tim Key from the Cancer Research UK and the University of Oxford states, "This decision doesn't mean you need to stop eating any [...] processed meat, but if you eat lots of it, you may want to think about cutting down. Eating bacon every once in a while isn't going to do much harm — having a healthy diet is all about moderation."

Conventional Meats: What do we mean by that? Conventional meats are those raised on farms where the animals are given antibiotics and/or hormones. This may include beef, chicken, other fowl, and pork; essentially non-organic, non-pastured, non-grass fed. Often, these animals are also fed feeds that are not "natural" for them to be consuming. All of these issues lead to major toxins and illnesses, not only in the animals, but in humans as well.

Antibiotics are often given to animals. Although antibiotics may help prevent active disease, these animals are not as healthy for us to eat. One major problem is that the antibiotics are passed onto humans. This can lead to resistant strains of bacteria. We do NOT want to be ingesting antibiotics when they are not needed. These antibiotics can also be passed into our drinking water through ground water and soil that is laden with animal excrement.

Antibiotics are used to keep animals free of disease, which allows them to grow more rapidly, gain weight, and be processed quicker. The consumer benefits because these cuts of meat are cheaper. It definitely is more expensive to buy organic and antibiotic-free meat, but the cost is certainly worthwhile. Why would animals need antibiotics in the first place? Because they are not being allowed to roam freely and are literally cooped up. Being in close quarters leads to illness and increases bacterial exposure. And as we shall see, eating the wrong diet can also increase animals' risk of sickness.

Hormones are a different story, but they can also affect humans. This primarily applies to beef. In the 1950s the FDA approved the use of hormones in beef cattle to increase the animals' growth rate and the efficiency by which they convert the feed they eat into meat. These hormones include natural estrogen, progesterone, testosterone, and their synthetic versions. One of the dangers is for pre-pubescent boys and girls. A 2009 study found that children who consumed the most protein from these animal sources entered puberty about seven months earlier than those who consumed the least. The concern becomes, what does beef injected with hormones do to the hormones of humans who consume them? Is there a link between consumption and hormonal-based cancers like breast, ovarian, and prostate?

Well, "red meat" does have its share of associations with cancer. The same review of studies by the IARC that found causation between cured meat and cancer also found that red meats "likely" cause cancer. This encompasses beef, lamb, and pork. *Overconsumption* of these can lead to issues. It's been positively associated with risk of cancers of the colon and rectum, esophagus, liver, lung, and pancreas. Experts agree, however, that meat is fine in moderation. Cancer Research UK states, "It's a good source of some nutrients such as protein, iron and zinc. It's just about being sensible, and not eating too much, too often."

Animal feeds are yet another story. By nature, cows were meant to eat grass. They are ruminants. This means they acquire nutrients in their specialized digestive tracts, first by fermenting the foods they eat in their stomach. In fact, their stomachs consist of four chambers to help with this fermentation. They eat food, often indigestible at first, regurgitate it, and then chew that cud again until it's broken down. When cows eat grains or corn and not the roughage they should, it forms a layer of foamy slime in their stomach called the rumen. This slime makes their stomachs acidic. Acidotic animals tend to have diarrhea, ulcers, bloating, liver disease, and a general weakening of the immune system. This makes them unhealthy. This is why antibiotics are administered, creating a vicious cycle.

Likewise, chickens are often given feeds unnatural to them. Pasture-raised chickens forage for seeds, green plants, and insects. Most caged chickens eat GMO feed (corn, soy, grains) containing pesticides, herbicides, and fungicides with little or no nutritional value. They, too, become sick. Think about it ... when humans eat nutritionally poor foods, they become ill. So too do animals. We don't want to eat sick animals. Remember, you are what you eat.

Farmed Fish: Farmed fish are different from wild caught fish. Farmed fish are actually grown in pens that are often submerged in ponds, lakes, or salt water. Wild caught fish, on the other hand, are fished from their natural environments. Due to the crowded conditions in which farmed fish live, they are given antibiotics to stave off diseases. The same problem applies as with conventional meat ... these antibiotics lead to resistant strains of bacteria. Humans are the ones that suffer from these infections. Fish farmers also treat their fish with pesticides to combat sea lice. Studies by the Environmental Working Group have found that cancer-causing polychlorinated biphenyls (PCBs) exist in farm-raised salmon at 16 times the rate of wild salmon. Polybrominated diphenyl ether (PBDE) is also found in farmed fish feed. PBDE is a known endocrine disruptor and thought to contribute to cancer. Another study, conducted at the University of New York at Albany found that dioxin levels in farm-raised salmon are 11 times higher than those in wild salmon. The WHO labels dioxins as one of the "dirty dozen" because they are highly toxic carcinogens and are stored for a long time in the body.

2) High Protein Diets

So this one is tricky too. Protein is a macronutrient. You need some in your diet because our body uses it to build and repair tissues. You also use protein to make enzymes, hormones, and other body chemicals. It is an important building block of bones, muscles, cartilage, skin, and blood. However, high amounts of protein may not be beneficial and are associated with cancer risk. (To clarify, we are referring to animal protein, not proteins found in vegetables or other foods.) Large amounts of protein are associated with elevated Insulin-Like Growth Factor (IGF). IGF not only affects the growth of healthy cells, but can also encourage cancer cell growth.

In a 2014 study published in the journal *Cell Metabolism*, more than 6,000 people over age 50 were studied. Respondents aged 50-65 reporting high protein intake had a 75% increase in overall mortality and a 4-fold increase in cancer death risk during the following 18 years. However, interestingly, high protein intake was associated with reduced cancer and overall mortality in respondents over 65. So, it appears that low protein intake during middle age followed by moderate to high protein consumption in older adults (over 65) may optimize health span and longevity.

Protein intake and its effect on the body is certainly complex. The WHO recommends people should generally stick with plant-based proteins and/or stay as close as possible to 0.36 grams of protein per pound of body weight per day. This is about 54 grams of protein per day for a 150-pound person.

To give you an example, 50 grams of protein would be 3 ounces of chicken breast plus 3 ounces of ground beef. Another example could be 3 ounces of turkey breast and a cup of Greek yogurt. Valter Longo, one of the authors of the study states, "Almost everyone is going to have a cancer cell or pre-cancer cell in them at some point. The question is: Does it progress? Turns out one of the major factors in determining if it does is protein intake."

3) Saturated Fat

Read this carefully ... You do NOT need to avoid all saturated fat. In fact, the theory that saturated fat causes heart disease has been largely debunked. In 2010, the *American Journal of Clinical Nutrition* put to rest almost 50 years of incorrect and unfounded thinking that saturated fat caused heart disease. It pooled together data from 21 unique studies that included almost 350,000 people, about 11,000 of whom developed cardiovascular disease (CVD), and tracked for an average of 14 years. The data concluded that there is no relationship between the intake of saturated fat and the incidence of heart disease or stroke.

World renowned heart surgeon Dr. Dwight Lundell says the root cause of cardiovascular disease is from inflammation. In an article he wrote for *Prevent Disease*, he says, "The injury and inflammation in our blood vessels is caused by the low fat diet recommended for years by mainstream medicine. What are the biggest culprits of chronic inflammation? Quite simply, they are the overload of simple, highly processed carbohydrates (sugar, flour and all the products made from them) and the excess consumption of omega-6 vegetable oils like soybean, corn and sunflower that are found in many processed foods."

Okay, so saturated fat doesn't cause heart disease, but what about cancer? A study published in the *American Journal of Epidemiology* shows a connection between high intake of saturated fat and non-Hodgkins lymphoma. However, this study also found that by increasing dietary fiber, the cancer risk was reduced regardless of saturated fat intake.

There also appears to be some connection between breast cancer and saturated fat. In a European study of over 300,000 women over 8 years, researchers found that women consuming the highest intake of saturated fat had the highest correlation to developing breast cancer. The researchers called it a "weak positive association," however, and noted that it was most significant in post-menopausal women not using hormone therapy.

High-fat diets have also been associated with an increase in the risk of cancers of the colon and rectum, prostate, and endometrium. This was cited in an article in the *Journal of the National Cancer Institute*. Researchers found, on an international scale, strong direct correlations between fat intake and incidence or mortality from these neoplasms.

The take-away message is that saturated fat, in high doses, may not do you any favors. The research is not definitive on saturated fat, however. The research did not specify which type of saturated fat was being consumed. Was it from conventional hormone-laden red meat? Was it from avocado? Clearly the *type* of saturated fat makes a difference.

The pros of saturated fat are that it helps with satiety. Also, fat, especially from organic or grass-fed animals, is nutritive, containing fat-soluble vitamins A, D, E, and K. Coconut oil also is a saturated fat, and remember that coconut oil is anti-carcinogenic. It is of paramount importance to choose the highest quality meats or other carriers of saturated fat.

Breast cancer experts recommend getting no more than 30 grams of saturated fat per day. The Cleveland Clinic recommends consuming no more than 10% of your calories from saturated fat, about 22 grams. This seems remarkably low. Consider **your** overall diet. If you're eliminating most undesirable, cancer-causing foods, your saturated fat intake could be higher, especially if it's from grass-fed cows or plant sources like coconut oil or avocado. However, if you're more of a moderator, eating little bits of these potentially harmful foods (i.e., conventional meats, processed or packaged foods), then limit your saturated fat intake.

4) Eggs

Are you confused yet? Yes, eggs were mentioned in the chapter "Foods That Heal" since breast cancer risk seems to be decreased with consumption of them. However, if you're worried about or have a predisposition to prostate, bladder, or colon cancer, you may want to reconsider.

Remember, egg yolks are rich in choline. Choline is a micronutrient known for its role in fetal brain and neurological development. Pregnant women are often advised to get more choline because of its benefit to the fetus. It's also helpful for liver and muscle function and overall energy. We do need some choline, but too much may be toxic.

It is important to note that there is an association between choline and cancer. A study published in the *American Journal of Clinical Nutrition* studied 47,896 men. In the study population, choline intake was associated with an increased risk of lethal prostate cancer. Another Harvard study entitled "Choline Intake and the Risk of Lethal Prostate Cancer" found that those with the highest choline intake had a 70% increased risk of fatal prostate cancer.

Egg consumption is also associated with cancers of the bladder and colon. The World Health Organization (WHO) analyzed data from 34 countries and determined that egg consumption was significantly and positively correlated with mortality from colon and rectal cancers in both men and women. Also, in the journal *International Urology and Nephrology*, a study found that moderate egg consumption tripled the risk of developing bladder cancer.

So what about egg whites? Aren't they supposed to be healthier? Well, some experts argue that even the whites should be avoided. First of all, if someone has an allergy to eggs, it's typically to the proteins found in the egg whites. Also, the whites are a concentrated source of protein. For the same reasons that a high protein diet could be carcinogenic, the proteins in egg whites may be too.

So avoid eggs completely? You be the judge. Eggs do have great benefits in their vitamin and micronutrient content. However, if you are worried about cancer, limit your exposure to them. Have them once or twice a week or less. You can get the same benefits, the same vitamins and minerals, from other foods. If you do eat eggs, make every effort to eat organic, cage-free eggs from pastured hens.

5) Dairy

By now you might be thinking, "What the heck? Should I just become a vegan?" As my superhero loving son likes to say, "Not so fast!" If you'll remember, we looked at the probiotic benefits of yogurt and kefir, and we saw that organic whey protein is anti-carcinogenic. Whey is a protein derived from milk. Not all milk is the same, however, nor are its byproducts.

Conventional dairy has much to be desired. Traditionally, dairy cows are given hormones. In 1994, the dairy industry started using a genetically engineered growth hormone, rBGH (recombinant bovine growth hormone) on cows in order to increase and extend milk production. This, however, led to sicker livestock, which led to ... you guessed it! ... antibiotic use. Samuel Epstein, MD, a scientist at the University of Illinois School of Public Health and one of the top experts on cancer prevention, wrote the books "What's In Your Milk?" and "Got (Genetically Engineered) Milk?" In them, he talks about how milk from cows given growth hormone is qualitatively different and is "supercharged with high levels of a natural growth factor (IGF-1), excess levels of which have been incriminated as major causes of breast, colon, and prostate cancers."

By nature, milk contains IGF (insulin-like growth factor). Both cow milk and human breast milk contain it. It's what nourishes an infant and causes the baby to grow and develop. It's absolutely there for a reason. However, once infancy or early childhood has ended, both cows and human infants wean. They no longer need this growth factor to flourish, so they then gain their nutrients from the foods they eat. As we saw in the dangers of high-protein diets, IGF is associated with increased cancer risk. It is anabolic and is implicated in breast, endometrial, ovarian, prostate, and other hormone-linked cancers. IGF also activates enzymes responsible for the production of new blood vessels required by a growing tumor. This is angiogenesis. The opposite of what we want. Remember, half of a chapter was devoted to the benefits of anti-angiogenesis.

Not all studies are clear on a definitive connection between milk and cancer. An article published in *Nutrition and Cancer* in the 1990s reviewed an observational study of more than 3,000 cancer patients and 1,000 control subjects not having cancer. Elevated risks were observed for cancers of the oral cavity, stomach, colon, rectum, lung, bladder, breast, and cervix among those who consumed whole milk. Risk decreased by drinking 2% milk and were even greater decreased when subjects consumed reduced fat milk. This study was based on interviews by cancer patients and is observational, thus not proving causation, but it's certainly food for thought.

Another observational study out of Japan published in 2007, followed over 11,000 people over 10 years. Through questionnaires, researchers tracked consumption of milk, butter, and yogurt. Deaths from hematopoietic neoplasm (typically leukemias) were associated with consumption of butter. A "nearly-significant" association was also found with milk. Their findings stated, "The frequencies of butter consumption, and probably that of milk, were correlated with hematopoietic neoplasm, particularly from non-lymphomas." Again, we need to take observational studies with a grain of salt, but they are worthy of noting.

What about yogurt? The aforementioned study didn't mention yogurt as causative. It may be safe to assume that consumption of yogurt is actually protective, largely due to its probiotic properties. If you'll remember, we included yogurt along with kefir as beneficial fermented foods and dairy products. Be careful not to buy products with an abundance of sugar, however. And try to go for organic versions.

So, overall, what should you do? Should you limit dairy? You certainly don't need to avoid it entirely, but you should limit certain forms. Conventional dairy appears to do more harm than good. As with all other animal-based products, you should look for organic forms of dairy. Milk and dairy products from grass-fed cows are also preferable. Always, always choose the highest quality when it comes to consuming meat and dairy products. These are not the area to cut corners to try and save money. You can try and save money on other food products, perhaps by buying fewer packaged foods or eating more vegetarian or legume protein-based dishes. But do not risk exposure to carcinogens by eating conventional forms of these products on a regular basis.

6) Processed Oils

Many oils you find on the grocer's shelves have been heavily processed and are considered "refined." But, some oils are quite safe and are preferred because of their health benefits. We are referring to olive oil or coconut oil, for example. Olive oil that is unrefined uses olives that have been pressed to extract the oil, but the oil itself hasn't been filtered, heated, treated with chemicals, and so on. In other words, without getting too technical, it's in its pure state. Virgin coconut oil, processed without chemicals or high heat, is rich in medium-chain fatty acids that are quickly absorbed into the body for energy. Other oils that are safe to consume are avocado oil, red palm oil, and sesame oil. These oils are extracted easily and safely from the foods they come from without being exposed to high heats or chemicals. They are not rancid or damaged in the process of extraction. Many health experts even recommend cooking with lard, tallow, butter, or ghee (all from animal fats). They are stable when cooked and do not oxidize. If you can tolerate them and if you're not sensitive or allergic to dairy, cooking with them is safe. Remember, though, that if you're watching your intake, these animal fats do contain saturated fat.

Most Vegetable Oils: When processed or heated at high temperatures, oils become oxidized and damaged. These oils are dangerous to our health because during processing, free radicals are created. Most "vegetable oils" you find on store shelves fit this bill. The most common include rapeseed (canola oil), soybean, corn, cottonseed, sunflower, safflower, peanut, etc. These oils were practically non-existent in the early 1900s. Not until chemical processing was developed did these oils come to be. These oils are extremely difficult and unnatural to extract. Think about this. How many corn kernels do you need to squeeze to even see a drop of liquid fat? How about cottonseed oil? Do you eat cotton? Cottonseed oil may contain natural toxins and probably has unacceptably high levels of pesticide residues (cotton is not classified as a food crop, and farmers use many agrichemicals when growing it).

How are these oils produced? To start, many vegetable oils come from genetically modified (GMO) crops. The seeds are heated to very high temperatures, oxidizing them and making them rancid. They are then processed with a petroleum solvent to extract the oils. More chemicals may be added for color and to deodorize them. They are about as far from being in their "natural" state as possible.

These oxidized fats cause inflammation and mutation in cells. That oxidation is linked to all sorts of issues from cancer, heart disease, endrometriosis, and PCOS. They also contain a high level of Omega-6 fats. Remember, we want our food intake ratio to be largely skewed towards consumption of Omega-3s. Consuming these oils throws off that ratio. These oils are in an incredible amount of processed foods. Limiting consumption of processed and packaged food will go a long way towards preventing ill health.

Hydrogenated Oils: Hydrogenation is a process in which a liquid unsaturated fat is turned into a solid fat by adding hydrogen. During this processing, a type of fat called **trans fat** is made. You've probably heard the warnings to avoid trans fats. Here's why: Hydrogenated oils are known to increase LDL ("bad") cholesterol and decrease HDL ("good"). Also, because these oils are unnatural, the body was not designed to digest them. Such foreign substances often cause false immune responses which can lead to autoimmune conditions or decreased immunity and illness. Furthermore, they *block* the production of chemicals that combat inflammation, help nerve functioning, and balance hormones. The bottom line is, trans fats promote inflammation and negatively impact cholesterol levels. Inflammation is at the heart of cancer development. Hydrogenated oils are typically made from those we mentioned above: vegetable oils, such as soybean oil, canola oil, corn oil, safflower oil, and sunflower oil. Add to that shortening and margarine. They are used in baked goods and processed, shelved foods like chips, crackers, coffee creamers, etc.

Fried Foods: Fried foods are doused in high temperature, often boiling, oils. By definition, most fried foods are trans fats because of the oils they are cooked in. Just heating these oils can actually generate potentially carcinogenic compounds, and then known carcinogens like HCAs and PAHs form when muscle meats (like chicken or pork) are cooked in the oil. Deep-fried plants, on the other hand, can form acrylamide. Acrylamide is a toxic chemical compound naturally occurring in low concentrations in some raw foods. Toxicity arises when fats in those foods are cooked in high temperatures and become oxidized. Acrylamide causes inflammation and has been associated with endometrial cancer, ovarian cancer, lung cancer, kidney cancer, and esophageal cancer. In studies, fried foods have been directly associated with breast cancer, prostate cancer, colon cancer, pancreatic cancer, lung cancer, oral and throat cancers, esophageal cancer, and cancer of the larynx. Although they might taste good, there are certainly no health benefits in consuming fried foods.

7) Sugar

We could almost write an entire book on the ill effects of sugar consumption. There is increasingly more and more data showing that sugar is not only not good for diabetics, but it's also associated with illness and death from heart disease and cancer. It is, quite possibly, at the root of every illness.

To be clear, we are not referring to the sugars from fruits. Fruits, in their natural forms, are filled with fiber, along with the fructose. Fiber slows the release of insulin as well. Fruits are filled with a multitude of vitamins and minerals. Sugar, processed from sugar cane, is very different and is devoid of nutrition.

In foods, sugar can go by various names, and is often considered a "hidden" ingredient. Some other names for sugar in processed foods are: high-fructose corn syrup, corn syrup, evaporated cane juice, agave, fruit juice concentrate, brown rice syrup, barley malt, dextrin, dextrose, glucose, fructose, lactose, malt syrup, maltodextrin, and rice syrup. There are others as well, but these are probably the most common. You truly need to be a label reader, especially when buying processed foods.

What about sugar's role in cancer? We need not even list all of the cancers that may be caused by sugar consumption because it plays a role in all cancers. Sugar causes inflammation in the body. The *American Journal of Clinical Nutrition* warns that processed sugars trigger the release of inflammatory messengers called cytokines. Inflammation in the body leads to cancers, pain, autoimmune conditions, etc.

Eating sugar also leads to insulin spikes. Insulin leads to storage of body fat, and body fat is one of the sites of estrogen production in the body. Excess estrogen is a problem for women predisposed to estrogen receptor positive breast cancers. Insulin and IGF have also been linked to tumor growth and with cancers of the colon, prostate, and pancreas.

Cancer cells love sugar. Sugar feeds tumors and encourages cancer growth. Cancer cells uptake sugar at 10-12 times the rate of healthy cells. In fact, that is the basis of PET (positron emission tomography) scans — one of the most accurate tools for detecting cancer growth. PET scans use radioactively labeled glucose to detect sugar-hungry tumor cells.

As a double whammy, sugar suppresses a key immune response known as phagocytosis, the Pac-Man effect of the immune system. So not only does sugar feed cancer, it decreases our innate ability to fight off illness.

Dr. Robert Lustig, a famous pediatric endocrinologist and author of the book *Fat Chance: Beating the Odds Against Sugar, Processed Food, Obesity, and Disease,* says that sugar is a huge risk factor in the development of cancer. He voices his concern over sugar consumption and its link with various diseases. In a lecture he gave entitled, "Sugar: The Bitter Truth," he directly implicates sugar as a toxin and goes so far as to call it "poison."

Try to avoid sugar-laden treats and sweets and sugary drinks, including fruit juices, at all costs. Sugar is not essential in our diets. It does an abundance of harm and is not your friend.

8) Artificial Sweeteners

Although no definitive links between artificial sweeteners and cancer exist, the jury is still out on their potential to cause disease. Simply put, some newer generation artificial sweeteners have not been around long enough to have been studied extensively. Other older versions of sweeteners (like saccharin) have shown carcinogenic changes in lab rats but not necessarily in humans. That being said, artificial sweeteners have been associated with numerous health problems as well as digestive issues.

The first big "red flag" is that these sweeteners are artificial. They are man-made, not real food, and are derived from chemicals. They were created to give a sweet flavor to foods, beverages, and chewing gums without the calories and blood glucose elevating effects of sugar. But as we will see, each type of artificial sweetener does come with some possible physiological side effects for those who consume them.

There are different brackets of sweeteners, depending on their chemical structure. The following are basic categories with their brand name versions listed in parentheses. You'll also note that each comes with commonly reported side effects.

Aspartame (Equal, NutraSweet): Aspartame is made from a combination of two amino acids, phenylalanine and aspartic acid. You'll see warning labels on products containing this sweetener to avoid consuming it if you have PKU (phenylketonuria), a genetic defect that causes phenylalanine to build up in the body. Of course, this is a rare condition. However, more commonly, people have reported side effects after consuming aspartame. These include headaches, anxiety, arthritis, abdominal pain, nausea, irritable bowel issues, seizures, mood changes, and weight gain.

Sucralose (Splenda): This artificial sweetener is actually derived from sugar, as the manufacturers claim. However, it is still chemically altered by chlorine. Some side effects include head and muscle aches, stomach cramps, diarrhea, bladder issues, skin irritation, dizziness, and inflammation. A recent study showed that consuming sucralose can reduce healthy intestinal bacteria, which leads to poor digestion, and possibly even autoimmune conditions. In 2016, the CSPI (Center for Science in the Public Interest) placed sucralose in its "avoid" category based on a review of a medical study that found it could be linked to leukemia in mice.

Acesulfame-K (Ace-K, Sunette, Sweet One, Sweet 'N Safe): Ace-K is made from potassium salt that contains methylene chloride. It's often combined with aspartame or other sweeteners in food products. Reported side effects are nausea, headaches, mood problems, impairment of the liver and kidneys, problems with eyesight, and possibly cancer. The methylene chloride in Ace-K is likely the problematic component. OSHA (Occupational Safety and Health Administration) considers methylene chloride to be a potential occupational carcinogen as it is also used in things like paint strippers, adhesives, and metal cleansers.

Saccharin (Sweet 'N Low): Saccharin is the oldest sweetener, created in 1879. In the 1970s, saccharin was required to carry a warning label that stated it caused cancer in lab animals because studies had shown that the sweetener caused bladder cancer in rats. However, the FDA has since lifted that requirement. In 2000, warning labels were removed after scientists found that rats have unique proteins in their urine that interact with saccharin, causing bladder cancer. Human urine does not contain that protein.

Despite the lack of evidence to support saccharin consumption and cancer, some consumers still note unpleasant side effects. Side effects of saccharin ingestion include allergies, nausea, diarrhea, skin problems, and other allergy-related symptoms.

Besides some of the nasty side effects listed above, artificial sweeteners can actually *lead* to sugar cravings. Seems counter-intuitive, doesn't it? When our brains sense we've eaten something sweet but no calories follow, it gets confused and tries to seek out additional sugar *with* calories, looking for some nutritive value. It becomes a vicious cycle of craving sweets. Also, because artificial sweeteners are much sweeter than sugar, our palates then tend to prefer foods with extremely sweet flavors. This means that foods without sugar or sweeteners may not taste as good to us and certainly do not become our preferred choices. We opt for diet sodas over water and diet ice cream over a bowl of berries.

Artificial sweeteners may also lead to a slowed metabolism. Studies have shown these sweeteners may slow down your metabolism and even release insulin into the blood stream, even though they contain no real sugar. One study, conducted on rats that consumed artificial sweeteners, showed the rats ate more, their metabolism slowed down, and they gained an average of 14% of their body fat, all within about two weeks. Another study on the effects of artificial sweeteners on atherosclerosis found that daily consumption of drinks with artificial sweeteners creates a 35% greater risk of metabolic syndrome (high blood pressure and blood sugar, excess body fat around the waist, and abnormal cholesterol levels) and a 67% increased risk for type 2 diabetes. This demonstrates that artificial sweeteners do have an impact on insulin, brain chemistry, and fat-storing abilities.

Regarding artificial sweetener use in general, CSPI president Michael F. Jacobson states the following:

> *We recommend that consumers avoid sucralose, or Splenda, and we recommend consumers also avoid saccharin, aspartame, and acesulfame potassium [Ace-K]. That said, the risk posed by over-consumption of sugar and high-fructose corn syrup, particularly from soda and other sugar-sweetened beverages, of diabetes, heart disease, and obesity, far outweighs the cancer risk posed by sucralose and most other artificial sweeteners. Consumers are better off drinking water, seltzer, or flavored waters, but diet soda does beat regular soda.*

Sugar is still the worst offender when it comes to our health and susceptibility to cancer. That being said, artificial sweeteners are not great either.

We should briefly note another class of sweeteners that is neither artificial nor an actual sugar, and that is the category of **sugar alcohols**. Some examples of sugar alcohols are xylitol, erythritol, mannitol, sorbitol, lactitol, and maltitol. Sugar alcohols are naturally found in plants like berries and other fruit. The carbohydrate in these plant products is altered through a chemical process. These sugar substitutes provide fewer calories than table sugar (sucrose), mainly because they are not well absorbed by the body. Therein lies the problem. Gastrointestinal upset is common, and gut flora (good bacteria) may also be altered. Consuming sugar alcohols results in less calories consumed and less blood sugar and insulin response, but there may be side effects. Sugar alcohols also are commonly derived from GMO plants, so they may have that toxic burden as well.

Are there any **healthier sweeteners**? The good news is that, yes, some natural sweeteners are deemed a bit safer, especially since they are not artificial. If you're looking to sweeten your tea, oatmeal, or baked good, for example, you can try adding some raw honey or maple syrup. Although these can slightly elevate your blood sugar, they also do provide nutrients. Using them judiciously and sparingly, when possible, is the key. Other good alternatives include stevia (a plant-based sweetener), monk fruit, coconut sugar, dates, and some fruit purees. And the best part ...

these natural sweeteners can actually contribute to your overall antioxidant intake! Win, win!

9) Refined Carbohydrates

Refined carbs are just another form of sugar. Essentially, when we eat these products, they turn into sugar in our body and bloodstream. They do the same damage that sugary foods do.

We are talking about all of the processed and packaged foods, forms of sugars and starches that don't exist in nature. In addition to the table sugar mentioned above, other examples include white bread, white flour, white pasta, chips, pretzels, crackers, cookies, instant rice, instant cereal, boxed cereal, refined starches, pancake mixes, fruit juices, sodas, corn syrup, fructose, dextrose, etc. Truly, the list is endless. Just remember, if it comes in a box, it's probably refined.

So what's the problem with these carbs? Much the same as sugar, they spike blood sugar and then insulin through the roof. Remember that when our bodies have elevated insulin levels, inflammation increases. Inflammation leads to irritation, decreased immunity, and ultimately to illness and disease. The other problem is that once you begin eating these carbs, you just want more. You may find that after a blood sugar surge, your energy drops. You may also experience food cravings to restore blood sugar again. It's a vicious cycle. Stay away from these foods for the same reasons you should stay away from sugar. Plus, they too have little nutritive value.

10) Gluten-Containing Grains

This is not necessarily a warning for all people, but for those with celiac disease and/or a gluten sensitivity, this message is critical. Many people without gluten·intolerances can consume quantities of gluten without digestive issue. However, there are entire camps of nutritionists and doctors who believe no one should consume gluten because of the hidden and underlying inflammation it causes. We'll get to that in a moment.

Let's look first at what gluten is. Gluten is a mixture of proteins found in wheat and other grains. The word gluten means "glue" in Latin. Gluten essentially creates the gummy, sticky substance of dough that helps hold things like breads and muffins together.

Gluten is found in wheat, rye, barley, and spelt. It's also found in malt, brewer's yeast, soy sauce, some soups, some lunch meats, sauces and gravies, salad dressings, and beer. One must read food labels carefully to check for ingredients as it is often hidden. If a package says, "Gluten Free," it should not contain any gluten or byproducts.

Gluten is also used in many refined and packaged foods. Pretty much all crackers, cookies, and other baked goods not labeled "Gluten Free" contain it. These products, as we've mentioned, create insulin spikes and act as sugar surges in our bodies. That is not to say that gluten-free products are any better in this regard. Packaged foods are packaged foods. Many gluten-free products have just as much sugar and processed oils.

These cause inflammation and lots of it. But gluten has some particularly harmful qualities above and beyond the insulin-spiking factors.

So why is this little protein so controversial? Well, for people with celiac disease, this protein damages the lining to their intestines, creating illness, malnourishment, and pain. Even for the non-celiac, gluten is implicated in other forms of inflammation. It has been associated with things like intestinal permeability and digestive issues, brain fog, skin conditions, hormonal imbalances and infertility, depression, chronic fatigue, fibromyalgia, and increased susceptibility to autoimmune conditions.

Dr. William Davis, cardiologist and author of the best-selling book *Wheat Belly*, implicates gluten and the corresponding inflammation it creates in numerous diseases. In an interview with the blogger "Wellness Mama," he states,

> *Wheat was the underlying cause for an incredible array of health problems and weight gain [in my patients], and elimination was key to astounding health. And note that this was not gluten avoidance for the gluten-sensitive; this was wheat avoidance for everybody, as it was a rare person who didn't experience at least some measurable improvement in health, if not outright transformation. I now recommend complete wheat avoidance for all my*

> *patients, as well as anyone else interested in regaining*
> *control over health and weight.*

In his patients following a gluten-free and/or grain-free diet, he noted improvement in diabetes, heart disease, acid reflux, irritable bowel, Crohn's disease and colitis, migraines, arthritis, joint pain, sinus congestion and infection, asthma, edema, and rashes. Weight loss was also a notable and welcome "side effect" of wheat elimination.

As far as gluten and cancer go, research is in its infancy. For years, researchers have known that those with celiac disease have an increased risk for developing certain cancers. There are three types of cancer associated with celiac disease: enteropathy-associated T-cell lymphoma (EATL), non-Hodgkin's lymphoma, and adenocarcinoma of the small intestine. In people with diagnosed celiac disease, ingesting gluten promotes an autoimmune response attacking the small intestines. These attacks lead to damage on the villi, small fingerlike projections that line the small intestine, that promote nutrient absorption. When the villi get damaged, nutrients cannot be absorbed properly into the body. The only treatment currently for celiac disease is following a strict, gluten-free diet. Once the intestines are healed, cancer risk decreases dramatically.

For those with gluten sensitivity, newer research shows some connection between a mere sensitivity and cancer. The reason this is important to note is that **millions** of people do not know they have a gluten sensitivity.

An article in the journal *Medical Hypotheses* states that gluten may be at the root of lymphomas in asymptomatic and latent celiac sprue. This means that many are undiagnosed but still are susceptible to an attack from gluten.

In a large study out of Ireland, published in *World Journal of Gastroenterology*, researchers found more deaths from cancer, plus more deaths from all causes, in people they defined as sensitive to gluten. Gluten sensitivity was determined by a positive AGA-IgA or AGA-IgG blood test (meaning their immune systems were reacting to gluten proteins), but a negative EMA-IgA blood test (which is specific to the type of intestinal damage found in celiac disease). Men in the group had a significantly higher than normal risk for all cancers. The types of cancer were not consistent except for non-Hodgkins lymphoma. The risk of developing this cancer was not only elevated, but deaths from it were increased among the men and women. One strange but interesting finding, was that women who had gluten sensitivity were *less* likely to develop breast cancer, and all participants were *less* likely to develop lung cancer. Researchers aren't sure why, but it may have to do with an immune system response. To be clear, ingesting gluten didn't help ward off cancer. Having the sensitivity and immune response markers did. Finally, overall deaths, and deaths specifically from cancer, were increased in people with non-celiac gluten sensitivity. Again, researchers aren't sure why, and they recommend further studies to investigate.

Unfortunately, much more research needs to be done to determine causation and to find whether gluten may cause long-term harm or whether eliminating it will reap lasting cancer-preventing benefits.

So, should you be tested for a sensitivity? It's difficult to say. You could have absolutely no immediate symptoms when ingesting gluten but still be sensitive to it. You could try an elimination diet for at least three weeks (perhaps longer) in which you ingest no gluten to see if you feel a difference.

Another problem with gluten is that sometimes, in people who indeed are sensitive, there is some cross-reaction with other foods. Gluten exposure can cause something referred to as "leaky gut," or intestinal permeability, essentially damaging the intestinal lining. Ingestion of gluten triggers a release of zonulin, a protein that can break apart the tight junctions holding your intestines together. This allows particles and molecules from the foods we eat into our blood stream, creating a cascade of immune responses. So, you may also be reacting to other foods in the same way as gluten.

This is of personal interest to me. I wondered whether I was sensitive to gluten after being diagnosed with PCOS (polycystic ovarian syndrome). I read about a possible connection to PCOS and gluten sensitivity. I decided to be tested and went through a naturopathic doctor to do so. In fact, blood tests revealed that I did, indeed, have a gluten sensitivity, and that I also was cross-reacting to eggs. The proteins in eggs were mimicking gluten in my system, also causing an immune response. This was particularly alarming as I had no immediate overt reactions when I ingested these foods.

Many doctors and nutritionists believe anyone with an autoimmune condition should stay away from gluten. Dr. Amy Myers, author of the book *The Autoimmune Solution*, recommends staying away from gluten permanently if you have an autoimmune condition, especially Hashimoto's Thyroiditis. She states that at least 30% of the population has gluten sensitivity, and an estimated 99% of people with celiac or gluten sensitivity are never diagnosed. When we eat gluten, enzymes break it down. One of the peptides that results is gliadin. In normal digestion, the gliadin is absorbed. However, in those with gluten sensitivity, the enzymes identify gliadin as a foreign invader and attempt to destroy it. The problem is, other tissues and organs are destroyed in the process. Dr. Myers states, "This is why gluten sensitivity is frequently paired with autoimmune conditions and why those with celiac disease are at risk of developing a second autoimmune disease." As we will see in later chapters, the association between autoimmune disease and cancer is high.

So you could be tested for sensitivity or you could just eliminate gluten for a time. Some choose to eliminate it entirely from their diets. If you can, it's not unwise to nix it completely as your body doesn't need it, and it may be doing unknown harm. There are alternatives to gluten-containing foods and there are a myriad of non-gluten grains. Many foods containing gluten are refined and processed anyway, and as we saw earlier, may lead to increased blood sugars, which in turn, can lead to inflammation and cancer. If you can't give it up, at least try to limit gluten.

11) GMO Foods

GMO stands for Genetically-Modified Organism. This is a new organism, not found in nature, that scientists have created and genetically engineered, usually not for health or nutrition purposes. Raising any red flags? It should.

Creators of GMOs believe that, among the many theorized benefits, genetic engineering can deliver higher crop yields; drought, bug, and pesticide resistant crops; and improved flavor. These are some of the most notable attributes of genetic engineering.

The California Department of Food & Agriculture has estimated that GMOs are now found in nearly 80% of all processed foods. The four most common GMO crops are corn, soy, canola, and cotton, but GMOs are making their way into a number of other common crops like potatoes, tomatoes, sugar, rice, and conventionally raised dairy and meat (as the animals are given feeds with GMOs).

But what do GMOs do to human's health? More research is still needed. However, consumption of GMOs has been associated with food allergies, organ damage, nervous system disorders, and some types of cancer. Many of the GMO seeds are becoming pesticide-resistant as well, which increases the need for excessive chemicals. It may be difficult at times to tell whether it's the GMO product causing the problem or the pesticides used to treat them. At any rate, there are health risks.

There are anecdotal stories of children being adversely affected by GMOs. A friend's son, who is autistic, seems to be much calmer when processed foods with GMOs are removed from his diet. Jeffrey Smith, author of *Genetic Roulette: The Documented Health Risks of Genetically Engineered Foods,* has also found GMO foods to be especially harmful to children. He says that, due to their immature and permeable guts, children have a higher exposure to GMOs in foods. These macromolecules leak through their intestines into the blood stream more readily, making the children more susceptible to attacks on their immune systems. This can result in allergies to foods and also in behavioral and cognitive changes.

A report published in the journal *Environmental Sciences Europe* revealed a connection between GMOs and organ damage, especially to the liver and kidneys, in lab rats. The review, conducted by Gilles-Eric Séralini, professor of molecular biology at the University of Caen in France, showed that consuming genetically modified corn or soybeans led to organ disruptions, with male kidneys responding the worst. They also found that a number of second generation female rats developed breast cancer. This means that the harmful effect of GMOs were being passed down to offspring.

Although more research needs to be done to gather a definitive connection between cancer and GMOs, there does not appear to be any health benefits to eating GMOs. Why take the risk of ingesting potentially toxic chemicals?

Remember, we're trying to avoid processed, refined, and packaged foods as much as possible. However, when you are shopping for such items look for the Non-GMO Project's certification stamp.

12) Canned Foods and BPA

BPA, or bisphenol-A, is a chemical used to make a hard clear plastic called polycarbonate, some sealants, and thermal paper such as the paper used to print cash register receipts. Most metal cans are lined with a sealant containing BPA. Also some older water or sports drink bottles (typically made before 2012) and sippy cups or baby bottles (typcially made before 2011) contain BPA. Newer legislation limits the use of BPA but does not prohibit it. Items that contain BPA may have a #7 inside the triangle on the outside of the plastic. Other products to avoid may have #3 or #6 plastic containers because they have known endocrine disruptors. Plastics considered to be safer would have #1, #2, #4, or #5.

So what's the problem with BPA? A 2015 article in the journal *Medicine (Baltimore)* reviewed and summarized the current literature regarding human exposure to BPA, the endocrine-disrupting effects of BPA, and the role of BPA in hormone-associated cancers of the breast, ovary, and prostate. Researchers found that BPA is a typical xenoestrogen (synthetic material that has estrogen-like qualities), and its estrogenic activity is likely responsible for its roles in promoting multiple cancers, especially that of the breast and ovary. They also found BPA promotes proliferation of prostate cancer cells. They even found that fetal exposure could be linked to future cancers.

At this time, the FDA does not consider BPA to be carcinogenic or harmful to human health. They argue that the trace amounts of chemicals that enter the body are rapidly metabolized and eliminated. The FDA states that studies that have assessed BPA provide no convincing evidence.

BPA, like any other potentially harmful substance, is best consumed in small quantities. There are ways to avoid unnecessary exposure to BPA. Look for plastics that have numbers known to be safe. If possible, buy fresh or frozen food products instead of canned. Glass jars or cardboard packaging are also preferable. Use glass or steel water bottles. Heat food in glass or ceramic containers, not in plastic. Wash your hands after handling receipts.

13) Alcohol

We do know that red wine is anti-angiogenic due to its polyphenols, especially resveratrol. Also in the chapter on cancer-preventative foods, we saw that some alcohol may be beneficial in warding off H. pylori infections, which could lead to stomach cancer. So, there are some benefits. However, alcohol consumed in large quantities and/or too often is associated with a greater risk for developing cancer.

In its 2016 *Report on Carcinogens*, The U.S. Department of Health and Human Services lists consumption of alcoholic beverages as a *known* carcinogen. The research evidence indicates that the more alcohol a person drinks, particularly the more alcohol a person drinks regularly over time, the higher his or her risk of developing an alcohol-associated cancer. A clear association exists between the following cancers and alcohol.

Head and Neck Cancer: This includes, but is not limited to, oral, throat, and laryngeal (voice box) cancers. Anyone consuming three or more drinks per day is at two to three times greater risk of developing one of these. That risk multiplies if the person also smokes or chews tobacco.

Esophageal Cancer: A 2008 study published in *BMC Cancer* found that drinking hard-liquor increased the risk of developing cancer of the esophagus. A low consumption of wine did not have the same effect. Like other cancers, the risk of developing this cancer also increases if a person smokes.

Lung Cancer: Another 2007 study found that drinking beer is associated with lung cancer increases. Researchers found that average beer consumption of one drink or more per day was associated with this risk of cancer. It was seen in both men and women but was significant in men.

Liver Cancer: As you well know, our livers filter toxins from our bodies. You probably know there is an association between alcohol and cirrhosis of the liver. Well, association also exists between alcohol and cancer of the liver. A meta-analysis of 112 publications was completed in 2015. Those who studied the literature found that one alcoholic drink per day was associated with an increased risk of developing liver cancer.

People infected with Hepatitis B or C also have an inherent increased risk and should not drink alcohol at all.

Breast Cancer: Many completed studies have shown links between alcohol and breast cancer. In a meta-analysis of 53 of those studies, researchers found that breast cancer risk increases with increasing consumption of alcohol. Women who drank more than three alcohol beverages per day were one and a half times more likely to develop breast cancer. For every glass of alcohol, risk increased by 7%. So consuming even one drink per day puts a woman at greater odds of developing the disease.

Colorectal Cancer: Studies have examined the correlation between alcohol consumption and colorectal cancer. Researchers found that people who regularly drank 50 or more grams of alcohol per day (approximately three and a half drinks) had one and a half times the risk of developing colorectal cancer as nondrinkers or occasional drinkers.

Alcohol is carcinogenic for a few reasons. First, the ethanol in alcoholic drinks must be metabolized and broken down. It then becomes acetaldehyde which is a known toxin and damages DNA and proteins. Alcohol also impairs our body's ability to absorb important vitamins and nutrients, especially vitamins A, C, D, E, and folate. It also increases blood levels of estrogen, which in excess, is known to increase risk for breast cancer and other hormonal cancers.

If you choose to drink, red wine is favorable. And with any alcohol, limit your intake to no more than an average of one drink per day or less.

If you have a personal or family history of the aforementioned cancers, it may be best to abstain completely.

14) Unfiltered Water

High quality, pure water is essential for every cell in our bodies. Clean water may just be the most important "nutrient" for effective detoxification and cancer prevention. Water helps to flush toxins out of our bodies. Our cells are also largely comprised of water, so proper cell function requires having adequate hydration. Research published in the *Journal of Clinical Oncology* reveals that water intake is inversely related to bladder, colon, and breast cancers; meaning the more water a person drinks, the less likely he or she is to develop these potentially fatal conditions.

Drinking filtered water is absolutely necessary when it comes to avoiding harmful chemicals or carcinogens that are often in regular tap water. Toxins present in tap water include the following: fluoride (yes, this is considered a neurotoxin), chlorine, lead, mercury, PCBs (chemicals used for industrial purposes), arsenic, perchlorate, dioxins, DDT, HCB (a pesticide), dacthal, and MtBe (a gasoline byproduct).

An article in *Environmental Health Perspectives* states that the strongest evidence for a cancer risk involves arsenic, which is linked to cancers of the liver, lung, bladder, and kidney. The article goes on to say, "The use of chlorine for water treatment to reduce the risk of infectious disease may account for a substantial portion of the cancer risk associated with drinking water." The article also notes that any and all chemicals generated by human activity can and will find their way into water supplies.

A report from the President's Cancer Panel on how to reduce exposure to carcinogens suggests that home-filtered tap water is a safer bet than even bottled water. This is largely due to the packaging which can leech BPA into the water. The Environmental Working Group (EWG) also found that pollutants still exist in some bottled water, possibly toxins that can even lead to cancer.

There are many different filtration systems, so do your research. The EWG has a good website (www.ewg.org) with recommendations on various water filters and the toxins removed by each. In general, however, a reverse osmosis filtration system is typically recommended. These can be purchased as a whole house system or an under-the-sink version. It gets rid of most contaminants, heavy metals, and other pollutants.

Choosing to drink filtered water, however you can get it, will help your body detoxify and also prevent new water-born toxins from entering your body. This is one of the most important steps you can take toward better health.

Final Thoughts on Foods to Limit or Avoid

If you're feeling like this chapter was all doom and gloom, please know that the information provided was not to scare you but to empower you, to help you make better choices. You certainly can still consume the foods listed, but now you know the facts behind why they may be harmful and why you may want to moderate or minimize your intake of them.

The good news is that you have choices. You don't have to overhaul your entire diet overnight. You can begin with some basic swaps like making baked potato wedges tossed in olive oil and salt instead of fast-food French fries that have been doused in hydrogenated oils, chemicals, and artificial flavorings. Begin with one snack, then make trades with one meal. Maybe for breakfast you make steel-cut oats topped with blueberries instead of your typical bowl of sugary cereal. Instead of your typical pasta dinner with a side of garlic bread, you switch to brown rice pasta with a side salad topped with avocado and seeds and dressed with olive oil and lemon juice. Instead of grilling multiple times a week, you decrease the amount of grilling and opt for easy slow cooker recipes. Use grass-fed beef or free-range poultry instead of conventional meats. Drink lots of filtered water instead of soft drinks. You can even sweeten that water if you like with flavored stevia drops or simply add some lemon or orange slices to it. Limit your beer and overall alcohol intake, but enjoy some red wine a couple times a week. Really, it's not so bad.

Sometimes it's hard to think of your health or future wellness when you're starving and faced with deciding on a quick dinner. As much as you can, try to be proactive and plan your meals. Try to remember that every little bit counts. Celebrate your small victories when you make good food choices. Try as best as you can to stay on track each day so that when you do indulge, you can enjoy those indulgences knowing that your overall diet nourishes you and will help you ward off disease and illness.

---

* Anticancer Action *

Remove as many packaged and processed foods as possible from your pantry, especially those with added sugars. From now on, don't buy any product that has more than 10 grams of sugar per serving.

Chapter 4: Vitamins & Supplements to Consider

We need to start by saying, you cannot supplement your way out of a bad diet. If you're eating a diet high in sugars, processed foods, conventional meats, and hydrogenated oils, no amount of supplements are going to be of real help. However, because even the healthiest eater may be missing some key nutrients, supplements can help to bridge the gap between a mostly healthy diet and a disease-free body.

Supplements can help us make sure we are getting the vitamins, minerals, and micronutrients our bodies need to function optimally. In fact, some supplements are proven to help with immunity and even to be anti-carcinogenic. Cancer is thought to be caused, in part, by nutrient deficiencies, so making sure you are not deficient in anything is part of the battle.

We will list quite a few supplements with their noted benefits. Know that many may be included in multivitamins. However, a word of caution regarding multivitamins ... not all are created equal. Some multis contain subpar forms of vitamins that are cheaper and less absorbable. We'll address these as we look at them. Some vitamins are also so essential and helpful that the quantities in multivitamins are less than the desirable amount, so these may need to be taken in stand-alone form additionally.

Other supplements we'll review are known anti-inflammatories or are known to be cancer preventative. Some are derived from herbs. Some are in the early stages of research but show promising signs for immune support. Let's dive in and explore the current research.

1) Vitamin C

We all know that vitamin C helps your immune system. You always hear of people drinking their orange juice and popping extra vitamin C when they're sick. There are certainly reasons why this is a good idea. An article in *The American Journal of Clinical Nutrition* reviewed more than 45 studies in which vitamin C was found to be protective against cancer. At least 70% of the studies found statistically significant protection, with high intake conferring approximately a twofold protective effect compared with low intake of vitamin C. They also assessed fruit intake and found that there were decreased risks for multiple cancers in those who consumed fruit rich in vitamin C. Those cancers were esophageal, laryngeal, oral, pancreatic, stomach, rectal, breast, cervical, and lung.

So eat your **fruits and vegetables**. Make sure your multivitamin contains at least **65-90 mg** of vitamin C. However, you can supplement with additional vitamin C. The upper recommended dose is **2,000 mg**, however it's almost impossible to "overdose." Taking too much vitamin C typically just results in nausea and/or diarrhea.

2) Vitamin D

Vitamin D is one of the nutrients people are most deficient in. **Vitamin D3** is the form that is most absorbable and should be taken.

Make sure your multivitamin contains D3 and not D2. Because it is so important and also because the general population is so often deficient, it's actually recommended to take additional vitamin D3 as a stand-alone supplement. **Actually the best source of vitamin D is the sun.** Getting a bit of daily sun exposure (10-15 minutes) is the best medicine. However, because we live in a society that spends most of its time indoors, supplementation is critical.

This vitamin is crucial for maintaining the health of the immune system. It's also important for strong bones and teeth, the cardiovascular system, and the neurologic system. Vitamin D is extremely important for regulating cell growth and for cell-to-cell communication. Some studies have suggested that calcitriol (the hormonally active form of vitamin D) can reduce cancer progression by slowing the growth and development of new blood vessels in cancerous tissue, increasing cancer cell death, and reducing metastases. The cancers for which the most human data are available are colorectal, breast, prostate, and pancreatic.

There is scientific evidence which shows you can decrease your risk of cancer by more than half simply by optimizing your vitamin D levels. Your serum level should hold steady at 50-70 ng/ml, but if you are worried about cancer, it should be closer to 80-90 ng/ml for optimal benefit. The dosage for supplementation would be based on your current serum blood levels. You'll need to work with your doctor to determine what your levels are and how much to include in your supplement regimen. However, given that so many are deficient, supplementing with at least **2,000 IU** is recommended for most people.

There is one caveat that most are unfamiliar with ... if you take vitamin D, you should also be taking vitamin K2. We'll discuss K2 next, but you need it to make sure vitamin D and calcium are doing what they should in the body.

3) Vitamin K2

As we just mentioned, vitamin K2 is an often overlooked vitamin and many are unaware of its benefits in the body. It is important to note that K2 *is NOT* the same as vitamin K1. Vitamin K1 (phylloquinone) is most often associated with green leafy vegetables. It is abundant in plant matter. People taking anticoagulants such as Coumadin are often advised to avoid consuming too much K1 because it works to clot blood and prevent excessive bleeding in the body.

Vitamin K2 (menaquinone), however, is found in **animal products like organ meats, dairy, and egg yolks**. It is also found abundantly in **natto**, a fermented soy-based dish popular in Japan. Interesting to note, meat, organs, and dairy from grass-fed beef contain much greater quantities of K2 than grain-fed beef. This is because the animal is designed to convert K1 from grasses to K2, a process that humans are ill-equipped to replicate.

Deficiencies in vitamin K2 are linked with cardiovascular disease, including artery calcification, osteoporosis, dental cavities and decay, decreased brain function, and cancer growth. Much of the issue with K2 deficiency has to do with its role in the absorption and use of vitamin D and calcium in the body.

We mentioned earlier that K2 and vitamin D work synergistically in the body. It is important to incorporate vitamin K2 into your supplement regimen because, without adequate K2, both calcium and vitamin D are ill-absorbed or, when absorbed, are transported to the wrong places.

Let's dive further ... When taken alone, calcium does not directly deposit into bones and teeth as once thought, but it can deposit into soft tissues and the vascular system. Aberrant calcium metabolism can lead to osteoporosis and heart disease. In order for calcium to make its way into the skeleton, osteocalcin production must be activated in the body. Osteocalcin is needed to bind calcium to the bone matrix. It is vitamin K2 that activates osteocalcin and directs calcium into the bones. Vitamin D helps the body then absorb the calcium that it acquires. If it isn't absorbed correctly, that calcium can end up in blood vessels, creating plaque.

Okay, so now we understand that we need K2 for heart and bones. What about cancer? A study published by the *European Prospective Investigation into Cancer and Nutrition (EPIC)* revealed that increased intake of vitamin K2 may reduce the risk of prostate cancer by 35%. Another unique mechanism of vitamin K2, demonstrated in bile duct cancers and leukemia, is autophagy, in which cancer cells essentially eat themselves by releasing their own digestive enzymes internally. By still another mechanism, vitamin C and K2 in combination contribute to cancer cell death by autoschizis. This is when cells simply split open, spilling their contents. Vitamin K2 also blocks new blood vessel formation that is essential to support the rapid growth of tumors (angiogenesis). Vitamin K2 has been studied and proven beneficial in the prevention of liver, bladder, and lung cancers as well, largely by the aforementioned mechanisms.

Dr. Kate Rhéaume-Bleue, N.D., author of the book *Vitamin K2 and the Calcium Paradox: How a Little-Known Vitamin Could Save Your Life*, recommends taking between **180 and 360 mcg** (micrograms) of K2 per day. This is more than the average American gets in his or her diet. She recommends taking 100 mcg of vitamin K2 for every 1,000 IU of vitamin D. So, for example, if you take 2,000 IU of vitamin D3, you should take about 200 mcg of vitamin K2. Also, taking **vitamin K2 in the form MK-7** is preferable due to its better absorption and longer half-life in the body.

4) Calcium

We need to mention calcium next since we just spoke about its synergistic relationship with vitamins D3 and K2. Your body needs calcium to build and maintain strong bones. Your heart, muscles, and nerves also need calcium to function properly. Some studies suggest that calcium, along with vitamins D and K, may have benefits beyond bone health: protecting against cancer, diabetes, and high blood pressure.

Which cancers appear to be reduced the most? Participants in the Nurses' Health Study who consumed more than 700 mg of calcium per day had up to a 45% reduced risk of colon cancer than those who consumed 500 mg or less per day. Also, Dartmouth Medical School researchers tracked 822 people who took either 1,200 mg of calcium every day or a placebo. Those who took calcium faithfully for four years had a 36% reduction in the development of new precancerous colon polyps five years after the study had ended. An article in *Breast Cancer Research and Treatment* also reviewed more than 35 studies which indicated strong evidence that vitamin D and calcium have a chemopreventive effect against breast cancer.

Dr. Rhéaume-Bleue, whom we mentioned in regard to vitamin K2, actually prefers that her patients **get calcium through foods versus supplements** since our diets typically provide us with what is needed. We know that **dairy** is full of calcium. For example, one glass of milk contains about 300 mg of calcium. However, if you are sensitive to dairy or are avoiding it, you'll need to get it elsewhere. Foods rich in calcium, besides dairy, are **white beans, canned salmon or sardines (with the bones), bok choy, kale, turnip greens, almonds, figs, or sesame seeds** to name a few.

If you do need to supplement, taking about **500-700 mg** of calcium per day is recommended. **Calcium citrate** is an absorbable form and is preferred to the cheaper, less bioavailable calcium carbonate.

5) Magnesium

Like calcium, magnesium is a mineral and also helps with the absorption of calcium and vitamin D. Without magnesium, calcium may be not fully utilized, and under-absorption problems (like arterial calcification or osteoporosis) may occur. When balancing calcium and magnesium, also keep in mind that vitamins K2 and D3 need to be considered. These four nutrients perform an intricate dance together, with one supporting the other.

Magnesium is the most commonly deficient mineral in people's diets. It's estimated that 80% of Americans do not have adequate serum levels of magnesium.

It is found abundantly in such foods as **green leafy vegetables, brown rice, oat bran, and lima beans**. Perhaps our less than desirable Western diets lead us to deficiency as packaged foods, flours, and sugars contain very little. Another theory is that we don't absorb magnesium from food easily, perhaps due to phytates in foods that bind to magnesium which then causes it to be excreted. Also, drinking soda, caffeine, and/or alcohol is known to leach magnesium from the body. If the city in which you live has soft water or if you have a water softener in your home, your drinking water likely contains much less magnesium than it should. Taking too much calcium can also lower magnesium levels. We need either a 1:1 or a 2:1 ratio of calcium to magnesium. For example, if you take 800 mg of calcium, you need at least **400 mg** of magnesium to counter-balance it. This is one mineral that most doctors and nutritionists advise taking as a stand-alone supplement in addition to the amount in your multivitamin. The most absorbable forms are **magnesium glycinate, malate, chloride, carbonate, or taurate**. Magnesium citrate can cause a laxative effect, so take caution if supplementing with that version

Magnesium is needed by every cell in the body, so it's truly important to make sure you're getting enough. It is essential for good sleep, as it is the relaxation mineral. Magnesium is also found in more than 300 different enzymes in your body and plays a role in your body's detoxification processes. Without it, our bodies cannot properly repair at the cellular level. In fact, healthy cells wither and die.

In a 2011 article in *Magnesium Research*, epidemiological studies identified magnesium deficiency as a risk factor for some types of human cancers. In addition, impaired magnesium levels were reported in cancer patients. A study published in the *American Journal of Clinical Nutrition* showed that higher intakes of dietary magnesium were associated with a lower risk of colorectal tumors. According to neurosurgeon and brain tumor specialist Dr. Russell Blaylock, low magnesium is associated with dramatic increases in free radical generation as well as glutathione depletion. This is important to note since glutathione is the "master antioxidant." Glutathione defends against free radical damage and also works to chelate (bind with and eliminate) cellular "filth" and any heavy metal toxicity, both of which can lead to cancer. So the health of our cells and immunity depends on adequate magnesium.

6) Zinc

I don't know about you, but when I think of stopping the common cold dead in its tracks, I think of zinc lozenges (Cold-Eeze is one brand example). Zinc helps with our immunity by potentially preventing the rhinovirus from multiplying. Rhinovirus is thought to be the virus associated with most common colds. Zinc also helps the immune system fight off other invading bacteria and viruses. It is a potent anti-inflammatory. In addition, the body needs zinc to make proteins and DNA, the genetic material in all cells. This is where more serious illnesses like cancer come into play because, as we know, cancer is essentially mutated and unhealthy cells.

A study cited in *Nutrition and Cancer* found that in patients with head and neck cancer, nearly 65% of these patients were zinc deficient. Zinc supplementation has beneficial effects on cancer by decreasing angiogenesis and increasing apoptosis (cell death) in cancer cells. Researchers stated, "We recommend further studies and propose that zinc should be utilized in the management and chemoprevention of cancer."

Zinc has also been studied and found to be helpful in the prevention of prostate and breast cancer. Interestingly, a 2012 study showed that even women with the BRCA1 gene mutation had a decreased chance of developing breast cancer if their zinc levels were sufficiently high. There is also an increased risk of bladder cancer and skin cancer with zinc deficiency.

You can get zinc in your diet through **oysters, red meat, poultry, beans, seeds, nuts, mushrooms, spinach, crab, lobster, whole grains, fortified breakfast cereals, and yogurt**.

When supplementing with zinc, it's important to take no more than 150 mg per day. Taking more than that on a regular basis is counter-productive and may do more harm than good. This is a conservative number as some naturopaths will tell you that you can consume much more. For a zinc deficiency, taking 50-100 mg of zinc daily seems beneficial. For a maintenance daily dose, opt for about **40 mg**.

Not all zincs are created equal. Different forms are available, but some are definitely better than others because of their absorption. **Zinc orotate** may be hard to find, but it is the best absorbed. Other good choices are **zinc gluconate** and **zinc citrate**.

7) Vitamin B12

Vitamin B12 is a nutrient that helps keep the body's nerve and blood cells healthy and helps make DNA, the genetic material in all cells. We need adequate B12 for energy. It also protects our heart, bones, nerves, and brain. Proper B12 levels help improve our mood and brain chemistry. And because it supports DNA health, it can help us feel and look younger and healthier. Its role in DNA synthesis and repair also makes it protective against cancer, as we will see.

The form of vitamin B12 you take is of utmost importance! Most multivitamins contain cyanocobalamin, which is a poorly absorbed and even detrimental (in large doses) form of B12. Especially if you are taking a stand-alone supplement, you need to look for **methylcobalamin**. Newer versions of multivitamins also contain methylcobalamin, so look for those next time you shop.

Why is methylcobalamin better for you? First off, cyanocobalamin is synthetic, even containing a cyanide group in its make-up (which has toxic effects over time). It is not the form found in nature. Our bodies have to convert it to a usable form. Herein lies the problem. A percentage of the population is not able to make this conversion. There are specific genetic mutations (MTHFR) that do not allow for this conversion. These mutations are actually more common than you may think. If someone has such a mutation, they cannot "methylate" or convert cyanocobalamin into its active form. This leaves free-floating, synthetic B12 in a person's bloodstream. This is a problem. Too much unabsorbed B12 has been known to *cause* cancer. You can be tested for an MTHFR mutation through a basic saliva test (23andme.com has an inexpensive one). But you really don't *need* to be tested. It's easy to just avoid the synthetic form.

So, **most people need only the amount of vitamin B12 (methylcobalamin) found in multivitamins**. However, to know if you are actually deficient in vitamin B12, you'll need to have blood work completed. Almost 40% of the U.S. population is deficient in vitamin B12 according to a recent study from Tufts University in Boston, and a vast majority of them are completely unaware.

A friend of mine, however, was extremely low in B12 and was quite symptomatic. She suffered from hand tremors, fatigue, and mild depression. She feared a larger issue was at play. But after having blood work completed, her doctor discovered low B12 levels and prescribed injections of the vitamin. Her symptoms then disappeared.

If blood work is not in the cards for you, at least take a multivitamin that contains the methylcobalamin form. If you are deficient, dosing will depend largely on what your current blood levels are.

Many vegans and vegetarians, especially, are deficient in vitamin B12. This is because the vitamin is NOT readily found in plant sources, but it is abundant in animal food sources. Also, if you are taking a proton pump inhibitor to reduce the production of stomach acid, you are also at risk for a B12 deficiency. This is because our stomachs absorb vitamin B12 through "intrinsic factor." When acid production is shut down, food and even vitamins are not broken down and absorbed completely.

Food sources rich in vitamin B12 are **yogurt, raw cheese and milk, cottage cheese, liver, grass-fed beef, lamb, sardines, mackerel, salmon, and tuna**. Fortified products like soy or breakfast cereal also contain B12, however be careful because "fortified" likely contains the synthetic version of B12.

How does vitamin B12 protect against cancer? A 2004 article in *Nutrition Journal* reviewed multiple experimental cancer studies carried out with various forms of vitamin B12. Researchers found methylcobalamin inhibited tumor growth in mice and caused mouse mammary tumor cells to undergo apoptosis (cancer cell death). In two prospective studies (one in Washington Country, Maryland, and the Nurses' Health Study) a relation between lower vitamin B12 status and statistically significant higher risk of breast cancer was found. Also, methylcobalamin, but not cyanocobalamin, increased the survival time of mice with implanted leukemia tumor cells.

8) Folate

Folate is another widely misunderstood vitamin. Folate is listed immediately following vitamin B12 because they often work in conjunction with one another. Folate is another vitamin that has a synthetic version toxic to some people, especially in high doses, and needs to be avoided.

Folic acid is the synthetic form. It is the form you've probably heard of and that is also widely found in cheaper, drug store multivitamins. Some newer vitamins do contain the natural form. (A quick search on Amazon will give you results and many options.) The form of folate you want to look for is **methylfolate**. Notice that, like the natural form of B12, it also contains a "methyl" group. For the same reasons synthetic B12 is not absorbed by many people, folic acid is not either. Those with a genetic mutation, again relatively common, cannot convert folic acid into the usable form of methylfolate in the body. And, like synthetic B12, too much synthetic free-floating and unabsorbed folic acid in the body actually is known to *cause* cancer.

Synthetic folic acid, in high quantities, has also been implicated as a cause for autism. A 2016 study out of Johns Hopkins followed 1,391 mothers between 1998 and 2013, following each for several years. They found that if folic acid levels in mothers were extremely high, as drawn shortly after giving birth, their babies' chances of developing autism doubled. Very high vitamin B12 levels in new moms were also potentially considered harmful, tripling the risk that her offspring would develop an autism spectrum disorder. If both levels were extremely high, the risk that a child developed the condition increased 17.6 times.

This is scary because folic acid is usually recommended by obstetricians to pregnant women. No doubt, much research has shown that adequate folate levels are protective against neural tube and other birth defects. Women just need to make sure they're taking methylfolate, especially in case they cannot properly convert folic acid.

So you can see synthetic versions lead to unabsorbed toxins which lead to various health issues. It's important to note that consuming the methylated versions of these vitamins, methylcobalamin and methylfolate, do NOT lead to abnormally high levels in the body because they're already in their natural and absorbable forms, and any excess can be excreted.

As for cancer, getting adequate folate is cancer protective. Many studies (listed in the same *Nutrition Journal* article mentioned above) have found a significant reduction in colon, rectal, and breast cancer with higher intakes of folate and their related nutrients (vitamin B6 and B12).

It's important to note that alcohol is an antagonist of folate, so drinking alcoholic beverages greatly magnifies the cancer risk of a low-folate diet.

You can get folate through natural sources especially **dark, leafy greens like spinach, collard greens, romaine, and kale**. Other good sources are **beef and chicken livers, brussels sprouts, sunflower seeds, asparagus, avocado, beets, papaya, hazelnuts, and sesame seeds**.

If you are pregnant or planning to get pregnant, it's essential to get adequate folate. Most doctors recommend at least taking a quality prenatal vitamin that contains folate. If you also supplement with extra folate, be sure to take methylfolate. It is advised that **women who are trying to conceive, pregnant, or breastfeeding get a total of at least 600 mcg (micrograms) of folate per day.** Some experts believe up to 1200 mcg is even better.

For the rest of the population, the recommendations are as follows: **Males over 13 years should get 400 micrograms; females over 13 years, 400-600 micrograms.** This is the amount found in most multi-vitamins, so taking a good daily multi should cover most bases.

9) Selenium

Selenium is a mineral that plays a crucial role in your cells' defenses against cancer. It is a central part of the enzymes that knock out free radicals, the unstable molecules that can attack your cells and ultimately lead to cancer. It also plays a role in recycling antioxidants through the body. These antioxidants, such as vitamin E, then lower the risk of cancer by preventing free radicals from damaging cells.

The *Physicians Committee for Responsible Medicine* states that studies have shown that selenium intake above the recommended dietary allowance (RDA), while not necessary for normal body function, may protect against certain cancers. In one region of China, where epidemic rates of esophageal and gastric cancers occurred, the risk was cut in half after large doses of selenium were given. In populations at higher risk for prostate cancer, selenium supplements decreased risk and growth rate of tumors. Selenium supplements may also be able to halt the growth of polyps in the colon and reduce the risk of lung and liver cancers.

However, it's still **best to get your selenium from foods** since it IS possible to take too much. The food with the richest source of selenium is **Brazil nuts**. Eating two or three nuts a day (that's it!) will help meet your daily requirement. Selenium is also known to boost thyroid function, so if you're someone who struggles with hypothyroidism, eat some Brazil nuts. Other food sources include **halibut, yellowfin tuna, sardines, grass-fed beef, turkey, chicken, beef liver, eggs, and spinach**.

While the U.S. RDA for selenium is **55 mcg (micrograms)**, studies show that for maximum protection against cancer, intake of selenium as high as **100 to 300 mcg** per day is necessary. Do not supplement with more than this, however, as selenium toxicity could occur. Signs and symptoms of toxicity include nail and hair loss, rashes, weight loss, fatigue, and irritability. Most multivitamins contain the RDA, so getting selenium through your multivitamin and food sources should be plenty.

10) Omega-3 Fish Oil

Omega-3 fish oils are considered essentially fatty acids. This means that our bodies need them but cannot make them. EPA (eicosapentaenoic acid) and DHA (docosahexaenoic acid) are the two main types and are primarily **found in cold-water fatty fish such as mackerel, sardines, salmon, herring, halibut, trout, anchovies, and tuna**. Salmon and other high Omega-3 fish obtain their dietary ALA (alpha-linolenic acid) from marine phytoplankton and seaweed and convert these marine plant sources of basic ALA into more useful forms such as EPA and DHA. Although we too can eat foods rich in ALA, we do not readily or fully convert those foods into EPA and DHA. Foods like flax, walnuts, chia, and hemp seeds contain ALA, but the human body doesn't easily convert these. Taking in already bioavailable EPA and DHA Omega-3 oils allows the body to use them right away.

Our bodies use Omega-3s to protect against oxidative stress and damage; support memory, learning, and mood; aid in maintaining a healthy immune system; support a healthy heart rhythm; help maintain healthy triglyceride levels; and promote the metabolism of dietary fats and cholesterol. As you can see, they help just about every body system.

It is important to have the proper ratio of Omega-3 and Omega-6 (another essential fatty acid) in the diet. Omega-3 fatty acids help reduce inflammation, and most Omega-6 fatty acids tend to promote inflammation. The SAD (standard American diet) contains way too much Omega-6. Studies suggest that higher dietary Omega-6 to Omega-3 ratios appear to be associated with worsening inflammation over time.

Omega-3s are excellent at reducing inflammation. They are often taken to help with ailments like rheumatoid and osteoarthritis, both inflammatory conditions. Remember, inflammation can take place anywhere in the body, and when it becomes excessive, cancers can also develop.

The University of Maryland Medical Center outlines Omega-3 fatty acids' role in prevention of cancer. They state that Omega-3s have been shown to help fight against colon, breast, and prostate cancers. The Eskimo population, who eat a diet high in Omega-3s and fish, have a low rate of colorectal cancer. Also, lab studies show Omega-3s prevent colon cancer from worsening. More research is needed in regard to breast cancer, however preliminary findings indicate women who eat more Omega-3s may have a deceased chance of developing cancer over time. Finally, population-based studies of groups of men suggest that a diet including Omega-3 fatty acids (from fish or fish oil) may help prevent the development of prostate cancer.

There is currently no official RDA (recommended daily allowance) for fish oil or Omega-3 EPA and DHA. Trying to consume fatty fish (like those mentioned above) several times a week is a great step. As far as supplements go, overall, most health organizations recommend a minimum of 250-500 mg combined EPA and DHA each day for healthy adults. However, higher amounts are often recommended for certain health conditions. **The dosages shown to be effective range from 200-4,000 mg.** Try to find a fish oil that has been third-party tested to be **free of mercury, heavy metals, and other environmental toxins**.

Be careful to not consume more than the maximum dose of 4,000 mg per day without working with a conventional or functional medicine doctor. In very high doses, Omega-3s can interact with blood thinners and aspirin, leading to excessive bleeding. It's also recommended to stop taking fish oil prior to any surgeries to decrease the risk of bleeding. Always tell your doctor if you are supplementing with fish oil.

As for food sources, look for fish that are lower in mercury. It is especially important for pregnant and nursing women and for young children to avoid mackerel, shark, swordfish, or tilefish because of their high risk for mercury contamination. Also, look for supplements that test for mercury and pesticide residues. You want to find the cleanest, purest forms of fish oil, especially when supplementing regularly.

11) Krill Oil

Krill are tiny shrimp-like creatures living in the world's oceans. They feed on phytoplankton, and are thus at the bottom of the aquatic food chain. Antarctic krill tend to be the coveted species for manufacturers because of the Southern Ocean's pure waters and the harvesting techniques. High quality krill oil is made by freezing the krill immediately upon harvest and then using a cold-vacuum extraction process to obtain the oils. This ensures that none of the nutritional value is lost upon degradation. Krill is thought to contain much less mercury than fish (and less contamination than some fish oils) because of its size and being at the bottom of the food chain.

Like fish oil, krill oil does contain EPA and DHA, albeit in lower quantities. These essential fatty acids provide the same benefits in krill oil as they do in fish oil. Krill oil, however, also contains phospholipids that potentially make them more absorbable. Fish oils, on the other hand, are attached to triglycerides which are thought to be less rapidly absorbed. Phospholipids (and the accompanying Omega-3s) are readily absorbed by the body because the cell walls in the human body are made from phospholipids. Arguably, krill is more "bioavailable" than fish oil. Because of the better absorption, less krill oil may need to be taken than fish oil.

Krill oil also contains astaxanthin. This is a powerful antioxidant and is thought to not only protect the oil to keep it from getting rancid or oxidized, but it works as an antioxidant in our bodies as well.

A 2016 study found that, in lab tests, extracts from krill oil were effective in suppressing colorectal cancer cells from forming and destroyed those that existed. Other benefits from krill oil come from its Omega-3 properties, just as those mentioned above in regard to fish oil.

As far as dosing goes, most people only need **two to three 500 mg capsules** of krill oil per day (each capsule typically contains about 50 mg of DHA and 90 mg of EPA). The pills are also much tinier and easier to swallow than fish oil. As with fish oil, look for krill oil that has been third-party tested for impurities. It's up to you whether you might take fish oil or krill oil. Some experts even recommend taking some of both, one for quicker absorption (krill oil) and one for the greater quantities of EPA and DHA (fish oil).

12) Cod Liver Oil

Did you ever hear your grandmother talk about taking cod liver oil by the spoonful? This oil has been around for centuries and used for its medicinal value by many generations. It went out of fashion after the advent of the daily multivitamin. But it's been given a resurgence lately as consumers drift back toward whole, natural foods and away from processed products and synthetic chemicals.

Like fish and krill oils, cod liver oil (CLO) contains Omega-3s in abundance. It is also a nutrient-dense source of essential vitamins including vitamins D and A. So, it is really a power-punch of nutrient density and provides the cancer-fighting properties in Omega-3s, A, and D.

A Norwegian study cited in *Anticancer: A New Way of Life* followed more than 60,000 women. It found that women who consume cod liver oil every day have 25% lower mortality from all cancers and 45% for lung cancer specifically.

There are different forms of CLO. You can buy it in liquid form, the traditional method. However, there are also companies that produce it in capsules. A popular version right now is a fermented form. The oils of fermented cod liver oil are extracted without heat, and preserved through a slow fermentation process. So the naturally occurring vitamins and goodness are retained. Some other CLOs, like extra-virgin cod liver oil, may also retain the naturally occurring vitamins. However, some forms of CLO require that the vitamins be added back in since heating during processing destroys them. You must read the labels to know for sure.

Fermented CLO and extra-virgin CLO contain the proper ratio of the essential fat soluble vitamins A and D, two nutrients that are neither able to be obtained through vegetable sources nor through some conventionally processed CLO supplements. And since these vitamins occur naturally and work synergistically in properly prepared CLO, there's no need to fear getting too much vitamin A.

Look for dosing on the label of the brand you buy. However, **1 tsp** is about the amount most recommend per day. Either a fermented CLO or an extra-virgin CLO would be best to find since we want to look for purity and do not want CLO thats natural vitamins have been eliminated through heat and processing.

13) Desiccated Liver

Here's a bit of good news. If you're like me and really can't stomach eating liver, taking desiccated liver tablets is a wonderful alternative. They have absolutely no disgusting taste to boot! We listed the benefits of organ meats in the chapter "Foods That Heal." Just to reiterate, liver contains vitamins A, D, E, K2, B12, and folate; minerals such as copper and iron; and Omega-3 fatty acids. It is jam-packed full of healing nutrients. We've previously discussed the importance of most of these nutrients in regard to their anticancer benefits. Each plays an important role. So, liver is one concentrated and amazing source of many cancer fighting agents.

When we speak of desiccated liver, we're primarily referring to beef liver. We also need to look for brands that are organic and grass-fed. We need to know the liver we're buying is pure and gives us the nutrients we need, not the toxins that may be filtered through the livers of grain-fed or hormone-injected conventional beef.

The brand I currently take is Perfect Desiccated Liver from grass-fed cattle. (I am not affiliated with this company in any way.) **Four capsules gives 3,000 mg of desiccated beef liver powder.** This is the company's recommended daily dosage. There are other brands available, of course. Just be sure to find desiccated liver **from grass-fed cattle**. There is no evaluation from the FDA regarding this supplement and no RDA (recommended daily allowance). However, remember it's truly not a supplement but rather a food that is dehydrated, powdered, and placed into capsules.

14) Hydrolyzed Collagen or Gelatin

You've probably heard of gelatin before, but hydrolyzed collagen (or collagen hydrolysate) may be a new one for you. Gelatin, of course, is the main ingredient in Jell-O (minus the sugar). Gelatin is a dried powder that's created from isolating and dehydrating parts of animals, including skin, bones, and tissue. That might sound pretty gross, but it's actually chock-full of amino acids which are the building blocks of protein. Bone broth, which we talked about in the chapter "Foods That Heal," is actually a rich source of gelatin. When you make bone broth, a layer of gelatin forms across the top. It can be skimmed off or consumed for an even healthier drink.

Hydrolyzed collagen is really very similar. In this form, the collagen is processed more intensively, which actually breaks up the proteins into smaller pieces. It is typically derived from bovine bone and cartilage. Usually, the bone is crushed, ground, defatted, soaked in acid to remove the calcium, soaked again to break the collagen bonds, and then dehydrated. This process results in small, intact amino acids which have not been damaged. These amino acids are quickly absorbed into the bloodstream, and are used as the building blocks of new collagen. Essentially, the amino acid content is the same as in gelatin, but the chemical structure has changed. Hydrolyzed collagen is easily mixed into liquids or foods without getting "gummy" because it's already been broken down.

So what are the benefits to taking gelatin or hydrolyzed collagen? First off, both are known for strengthening bones and teeth and for making skin and hair beautiful, largely because collagen is a building block for each of these body systems. Gelatin and collagen hydrolysate are also thought to help with inflammation in joints and the pain associated with that. Both are rich in amino acids like glycine. Glycine, for example, helps to repair our gut linings. When our intestinal walls are damaged, food particles and bacteria or yeast can enter our bloodstreams, creating food intolerances/ allergies and illness. Gelatin and collagen can also help to increase gastric acid which helps with absorption of nutrients in our foods. Without proper absorption, we are missing key vitamins and minerals even though we may be consuming foods rich in them. And probably the most important attribute is that these foods lower overall body inflammation. Reducing inflammation helps the heart and arteries, but it also lessens the chance of developing more serious illnesses like cancer.

In one 2003 study, researchers found that gelatin derived from pork suppressed human tumor cells in vitro (in petri dishes). The cancers tested were a form of leukemia, colon cancer, and gastric cancer. Another study in 2011 tested jellyfish collagen hydrolysate on mice. Researchers found that the greater amount of collagen hydrolysate given, the more antioxidant benefits the mice shared.

If you decide to add nourishing gelatin or collagen hydrolysate to your diet, you can find powdered forms on Amazon. I personally like the Great Lakes brand (again, I have no affiliation with the company). Great Lakes

Collagen Hydrolysate is from pasture-raised beef, so it's a great quality. **They recommend taking two tablespoons twice daily. Two T gives 12g of collagen hydrolysate and 11g of protein.** Because it is mixable, you can add it directly to water or coffee, etc. I put mine in my morning smoothie. The company also makes gelatin. This would be used more in making gelatin products like gummy vitamins, homemade jello, etc. **One T of this gives 12g of gelatin and 11g of protein.**

15) Turmeric/Curcumin

We previously talked about turmeric when we looked at anti-angiogenic foods. It is a powerful spice, known for its antioxidant properties. It is a member of the ginger family. Turmeric is used to make curry powder and is often in both Asian and Indian dishes. The main active ingredient is curcumin.

Turmeric Curcumin is also sold as a stand-alone supplement. This allows a person to get a hefty dose without having to cook with it. When taking this supplement, it is important to get a brand that includes piperine (or Bio-Perine). Piperine is an extract derived from black pepper and is what gives peppers their spicy taste. This extract has been found to increase the absorption of a variety of nutrients. It may also have immune-suppressing, tumor-inhibiting, and antidepressant effects. Without piperine, turmeric is not as readily absorbed. Piperine increases turmeric's bioavailability by 154%. (Likewise, if you're cooking with turmeric, use some black pepper to add to the absorbability.) In the brand I currently take, **two capsules contain 980 mg of organic turmeric**

root, 300 mg of non-GMO curcumin extract, and 5 mg of non-GMO Bio-Perine.

As for studies regarding anticancer properties of turmeric, research is in early stages. One phase 1 clinical trial showed curcumin could stop the precancerous changes in different organs. Some studies have also shown turmeric to be effective in helping to treat active cancers, especially the bowel and breast, when combined with other cancer therapies.

16) Probiotics

We already spoke about probiotics in relation to resistant starches, fermented foods, and yogurt. We already know that probiotics are beneficial because they inundate our bodies with healthy bacteria. Did you know that 80% of your immune system is actually in your digestive tract? It makes sense then that probiotics would enhance our immunity towards myriads of illnesses and diseases. Taking probiotics helps to ensure that our bodies are not experiencing dysbiosis, when bad bacteria overwhelm the good.

In 2010, the *International Journal of Food Sciences and Nutrition* stated,

> *Studies on the effect of probiotic consumption on cancer appear promising, since recent in vitro and in vivo studies have indicated that probiotic bacteria might reduce the risk, incidence and number of tumors of the colon, liver and bladder. The protective effect against*

cancer development may be ascribed to binding of mutagens by intestinal bacteria, suppressing the growth of bacteria that convert procarcinogens, [...] or merely by enhancing the immune system of the host.

In other words, probiotics can increase immunity and crowd out the bad bacteria.

Other studies have seen probiotics assist in recovery of cancer patients undergoing chemotherapy. They've also been shown to help decrease inflammation from cancer surgery. And lastly, they help to diminish the diarrhea that often comes with certain forms of radiation.

When looking for a probiotic, there are some important things to consider. Look for quality, reputable brands. **Look for probiotics with a high CFU (colony forming unit), from 15 billion to 100 billion.** Probiotics with multiple strains are also beneficial, since bacterial diversity helps to attack unwanted "bad" bacteria. Look for strains like **bacillus coagulans (and other bacillus strains); saccharomyces boulardii; lactobacillus rhamnosus (and other lactobacillus strains); and bifidobacterium bifidum (and other bifidobacterium strains).** These are just a few strains known to be beneficial and able to withstand digestion.

17) Coenzyme Q10

Coenzyme Q10, familiarly known as CoQ10, is a natural antioxidant which is, actually, innately synthesized by our bodies. It is also found in many foods such as **organ meats, beef, sardines, mackerel, olive oil, peanuts, spinach, broccoli, and cauliflower**.

CoQ10 is so important because it protects the body from the harmful effects of free radicals, thus reducing one's risk of developing cancer. It is found in every cell, and it is used to produce the energy needed for cell growth, maintenance, and DNA repair.

A few studies have shown low blood levels of CoQ10 in some cancer patients. These patients suffered from myeloma, lymphoma, and other types of cancer such as head and neck, breast, lung, pancreatic, colon, kidney, and prostate. It may be that a deficiency of CoQ10 is a common factor in the development of cancer, or it may follow that CoQ10 is depleted in cancer patients. Researchers are unsure.

CoQ10 has also been deemed effective when used as an adjuvant therapy for cancer (in addition to primary treatments like chemotherapy), helping to halt the growth of cancer cells. This has been demonstrated largely in laboratory settings. However, human studies have shown that CoQ10 does boost the immune system.

Supplementation with CoQ10 is often important because as we age, our bodies begin to produce less and less of it. A reduction of this coenzyme can lead to faster aging as well as various ailments, as mentioned above. Also, if you take cholesterol-lowering statins, your body becomes even more depleted in CoQ10, and it is essential that you supplement with it to avoid muscle aches, weakness, and possibly even memory loss.

CoQ10 comes in two forms: ubiquinol, the active antioxidant form, and ubiquinone, the oxidized form, which the body partially converts to ubiquinol. Ubiquinol appears to be slightly more bioavailable, so look for this form of CoQ10, and also look to get it in soft gel form for better absorption. **The general adult population should aim to take at least 100 mg of CoQ10 daily. If you take a statin or have existing heart disease, aim to take 200 mg per day.**

18) DIM

DIM stands for Diindolylmethane. It is a food-based compound found in **cruciferous vegetables like broccoli, cabbage, cauliflower, and Brussel's sprouts**. The body makes DIM from a substance called indole-3-carbinol (I3C), which is found in these vegetables. DIM supplements also are available from many retail sources.

The *Memorial Sloan Kettering Cancer Center* reports that studies have shown DIM has the ability to reduce the risk of certain cancers. Those cancers influenced by excessive estrogen levels, such as breast, cervix, uterine, and prostate, especially benefit from DIM supplementation. Colon, thyroid, lung, and other cancers may also be inhibited. DIM works by helping the body to make a better balance of the "good estrogen" (2-hydroxy-estrone) compared to the "bad estrogen" (16-alpha-hydroxy-estrone).

Researchers have shown that DIM is able to stop tumors from completing angiogenesis and creating their own blood supplies.

Moreover, the level of oxygen in tumor cells is increased by the use of DIM. Oxygen is the mortal enemy of cancer.

So why not just eat your veggies? Why supplement with DIM? Well, it would require eating about two and a half pounds of cruciferous vegetables to get just 25 mg of DIM. In contrast, a good DIM supplement will contain about **100 mg of DIM**. This amount is necessary to achieve the hormonal health we are after. Just be aware that doses in excess of this could lead to stomach upset or headaches.

A daily dose of 108 mg has been used in clinical studies with no significant side effects. Of course, if you take any prescription medications, discuss use of DIM with your doctor to determine if it is appropriate for your situation. Pregnant or lactating women should also avoid DIM since there are not enough studies to determine its effects on babies. Overall however, there are very little known side effects to taking DIM. Remember, this is a food-derived supplement.

19) Grape Seed Extract

We talked about grape seed oil in the anti-angiogenic foods section. The extract is essentially the same thing but can be taken as a supplement. It is usually sold as an over-the-counter product in the United States in the form of capsules or tablets (100-500 mg) and sometimes in the form of a liquid with dropper.

Studies have shown that grape seed extract is effective at inhibiting tumor growth in several cancers. Skin, colorectal, prostate, breast, lung, stomach, and oral cancers have all undergone lab studies. Grape Seed Extract (GSE) was found to induce apoptosis (abnormal cell death) and was found to be anti-angiogenic in those cancers.

In addition to being anti-inflammatory, GSE is also known for helping with poor circulation, high blood pressure, high cholesterol, and with swelling caused by injury.

If you decide to supplement with GSE, doses of between **100-300 milligrams per day** have been used in studies. This amount is also prescribed in some European countries.

20) Essential Oils

This is a very broad category. Because there are literally hundreds of essential oils, we'll just list some that are thought to be beneficial in the prevention and possibly even in the treatment of cancer. Please know that these are NOT intended to be used as a sole therapy to treat cancer if you've already been diagnosed. They may be an adjunct to other treatments. We'll also not go into detail on any one essential oil since there are many. If you're interested in learning more about essential oils and their impact on cancer, a good reference might be www.drericz.com which gives a comprehensive list.

The following is a list of essential oils thought to be helpful in regard to cancer prevention and healing. You'll note that several of these were also listed as beneficial spices and herbs previously.

* Citrus Oil

* Clary Sage

* Frankincense

* Lavender

* Lemongrass

* Myrrh

* Peppermint & Spearmint

* Thyme

* Sandalwood

* Balsam Fir

* Hyssop

* Orange

* Tsuga

* Black Pepper

* Cinnamon

* Clove

* Oregano

* Cardamom

* Fennel

* Rosemary

* Mistletoe

The website www.mindbodygreen.com suggests that some of these oils can be taken orally in a gel capsule by combining approximately seven drops of the oil with a carrier oil (like coconut oil, for example), and as dosage increases, can be taken in up to six capsules per day. They also note that the body can develop a resistance to one essential oil over time, so it may be important to alternate every three to four weeks the type of oil you use.

Again, please consult your doctor or naturopath before taking these oils, especially if you do already suffer from cancer. Because this is not a book focused on essential oils, this information is for reference only. You should do more research on your own and/or with your doctor if essential oils are something you'd like to consider.

21) Aspirin

Aspirin is not a supplement but a drug and should be treated as such. It is NOT for everyone to take, and there are certainly side effects if taken by the wrong person or by a person with a contraindicated condition.

Firstly, anyone with an active bleed or history of a bleeding condition should take caution. Aspirin works as an anti-platelet which helps to keep blood from clotting. This is what makes it useful in heart disease and to prevent stroke. However, if you have a history of ulcers, gastritis, gastrointestinal bleeding, or hemorrhagic stroke, you should avoid aspirin because it could exacerbate those conditions. Also, if you consume three or more alcoholic drinks per day, aspirin could cause serious stomach bleeding. There are also people who are allergic to aspirin and should not consume it.

Contraindications aside, aspirin does appear to be helpful in the prevention of certain cancers. Men who take aspirin or other non-steroidal anti-inflammatory drugs appear to have a lower risk of colon cancer and possibly prostate cancer. Also, a study from the U.S. National Cancer Institute found that women who used aspirin daily had a 20% lower risk of ovarian cancer than those who used aspirin less than once a week.

In 2012, a meta-analysis of 23 studies on aspirin therapy was reviewed in the *American Journal of Medicine*. The analysts found that overall cancer deaths were reduced by low-dose aspirin therapy.

Low-dose aspirin or "baby" aspirin (**81 mg**) would be the preferred method for prevention of any cancers. One could reap those benefits while lessening the chance for bleeding. Aspirin still needs to be studied in greater detail to definitively say there is any connection with cancer prevention. However, if you're taking low-dose aspirin for cardiac reasons, you may receive some added advantages. Again, please consult your doctor if you do choose to take a daily low-dose aspirin.

22) High-Quality Multivitamin

Probably the best thing you can do regularly is to make sure you're eating a well-balanced, whole foods diet. A close second is to take a good multivitamin/multimineral supplement. This will make sure you're getting an array of vitamins and minerals that might be missing from your diet.

In this chapter, we've looked at the harm caused by synthetic forms of vitamin B12 and folic acid. There are other vitamins, some of which we'll discuss in the next chapter, that also have synthetic forms and also appear to be harmful. So, it would do us well to choose a multivitamin that does NOT contain synthetic forms.

I have no affiliation with any of the companies I'm about to mention. However, on my quest to find the best multivitamin, I've found several that contain good quality, absorbable forms of vitamins with reviews from professionals that can attest to their efficacy.

Smarty Pants: These are gummy vitamins which makes them easy to chew and swallow, and they are yummy, too! The company prides themselves on their non-GMO, gluten-free, dairy-free, non-synthetic, etc. Their vitamins also contain Omega-3s as an added bonus. Best of all, you can now find these at most drug stores and grocers. Of this brand, I like the Women's Complete, Men's Complete, Prenatal Complete, Adult Complete, and Kids Complete. They also make probiotic blends and multivitamins that contain fiber. Since the product's conception, it appears the formulations have changed ... in a good way. The newer vitamins contain the methylated versions of B12 and folate.

Thorne Research: This company has a host of great supplements anywhere from sports performance amino acids to immune system boosters to weight management aids. However, for a multivitamin, I would recommend their Basic Nutrients 2/Day. They also have a few other "Basic Nutrients" blends that do or don't contain copper and iron. Take a look at their website to find the best one for you. Again, this company prides itself of providing the methylated forms of vitamins and high quality minerals.

Pure Encapsulations: This is another company that has a host of different vitamins and supplements to choose from. They, too, are sure to include non-synthetic forms of vitamins in their blends. You'll probably need to order from their website as they're not readily available in stores. Their multivitamin is "Multi t/d" (two/day). They also have a formulation just for men and one just for women.

Naturelo: You can find these on Amazon. The company makes a Naturelo for Men and a Naturelo for Women. The vitamins are whole-food based and made from organic ingredients. The forms are non-synthetic and the minerals have the correct balance/ratio. They also add in some foods-based, antioxidant blends for added health benefits.

Mary Ruth Organics: This company has its own website, but you'll also be able to order these through Amazon. A host of products are sold, but for multivitamin purposes, look for the "Liquid Morning Multivitamin" and "Liquid Nightime Multimineral." For better absorbency and to avoid counter-acting one another, the vitamins and minerals are divided up to some degree, thus a separate morning and evening formulation. The company prides itself on being vegan, non-GMO, gluten-free, dairy-free, soy-free, nut-free, organic, and without sugar or nightshades. (Nightshades are members of the tomato, potato, eggplant, and pepper families. These are avoided because many people have sensitivities or reactions to them.) No synthetic vitamins are used. You'll take 2 T of the raspberry/cherry-flavored multivitamin in the morning, and 2 T of the coconut-flavored multimineral at night. They can be taken by the spoonful or mixed into water or juice. They really have a pleasant taste.

Nutreince: The manufacturer, Calton Nutrition, came out with this powdered multivitamin which also has an AM and PM dose. The powder can be mixed with water or juice. It has a patented "Anti-Competition Technology" which separates competing vitamins and/or minerals for maximum absorption. It uses the most absorbable form of each micronutrient. The company's philosophy is that, since at the heart of most illnesses is a micronutrient deficiency, these powders will meet all the micronutrient requirements a person needs. Beyond just the typical vitamins and minerals, this multi also contains supplements like CoQ10, alph lipoic acid (ALA), carnitine, choline, quercetin, and grapeseed extract. The product is available through the Calton Nutrition website.

The above suggested brands are a starting point for you. Please do your own research and decide which multi is best for you. Remember to look for methylated and/or absorbable forms of vitamins and well as those that are non-synthetic, and, preferably, non-GMO. Final Thoughts on Vitamins & Supplements

Remember that supplements are a way of covering our bases to ensure we're getting all of the vitamins, minerals, and micronutrients we need to stay healthy. Many modern convenience foods contain little nourishment with hefty amounts of calories. It is possible to be fat and "starving" at the same time.

Even healthier foods like fruits and vegetables might not have the same nutritional value as those consumed by our parents and grandparents. Our soils are being depleted of essential nutrients. When plants are repeatedly grown on the same land, the soil loses vitamins, minerals, and microbes faster than they can be replaced. Over time, the plants have fewer nutrients to grow. Non-organic foods also contain fewer nutrients and cancer-fighting polyphenols, and we know that it's not always possible to eat organic.

We also live in a world surrounded by and inundated with toxins. By taking supplements, we're arming our bodies with the defenses they need to remain healthy, even when faced with potentially hazardous exposures.

Exercising can also deplete our nutrient stores. Of course, exercise is a great thing for our overall health and well-being. However, especially intense, sweat-breaking work outs or long-distance, long-duration training will result in an increased need for more nutrients.

One last note, as we age, our ability to absorb necessary vitamins and minerals declines. Hydrochloric acid and digestive enzyme production naturally diminish, making it more difficult to break down and absorb nutrients from foods. Also with age, many people tend to need more medication for various health issues. Medications can interfere with nutrient absorption as well, increasing the need for more nutrients. Supplements can provide that added boost to ensure there are no deficiencies.

So it seems that most of us can benefit from, at the bare minimum, a high-quality multivitamin and mineral supplement. As always, look at the ingredients to check that supplements are not loaded with fillers and sugars. Look for non-GMO products when applicable. Read the labels for dosing amounts. Be sure to list the supplements you take when you visit your doctor. It's important that doctors know your current supplement regimen to look for interactions with medications.

```
┌─────────────────────────────────────────────────────┐
│                 * Anticancer Action *                │
│                                                       │
│  If you're on a budget or just looking to narrow down the list of │
│  supplements, here are the top six I recommend with reminders why │
│                   they're so important.               │
│                                                       │
│              Begin taking these daily.                │
└─────────────────────────────────────────────────────┘
```

1) Multivitamin — A high-quality multivitamin, multi-mineral complex is of utmost importance to connect the dots in any missing nutrition in our diets. Be sure to look for methylated forms of folate and vitamin B12.

2) Vitamin D — So many people are deficient in vitamin D, and it is so essential for our immune systems to function optimally. Remember to buy it as the D3 version and aim for at least 2,000 IU per day.

3) Vitamin K2 — In order to properly absorb vitamin D and calcium, one must incorporate K2 into the mix. It helps prevent arterial plaque, heart disease, and cancer. You can find vitamin K2/D3 combination liquids on the market. If taking K2 separately, be sure to look for the MK-7 version and aim for 180-360 mcg per day.

4) Magnesium — Because it is THE MOST commonly deficient mineral in our diets, we need to take extra. We need magnesium for restful sleep, protein synthesis, nerve functioning, blood pressure and blood sugar regulation, and for detoxification ... to name a few. Look for magnesium glycinate, malate, chloride, carbonate, or taurate. Take 400-800 mg per day, and take it at bedtime to aid with sleep.

5) Omega-3 Fish Oil — It is an essential fatty acid, and we probably don't get enough in our diets. Omega-3 helps with cognitive function, immune support, and healthy heart and cholesterol levels. A daily intake of 1,000-4,000 mg is often recommended.

6) Probiotic — Probiotics help our immune system by crowding out bad bacteria with good bacteria. They help with digestion and absorption of vitamins and minerals. Look for a probiotic that includes various strains, and rotate your probiotics occasionally to help with bacterial diversity.

Chapter 5: Supplements & Medications to Limit or Avoid

Not all supplements are beneficial to our health. Some poor quality vitamins and supplements could not only be unhelpful but a waste of money. Others could build up in our systems, causing reactions. It's important to know *why* you are taking any supplements and whether or not you really need them.

On the other hand, even some medications can deplete our nutrient stores and can do more harm than good. One BIG disclaimer ... do NOT stop taking any medication you're currently on without consulting your doctor. However, some of the medications we'll discuss may be "optional," and it may be up to you whether or not to continue taking them. We'll also look at some medications that might have especially harmful side effects and/or are known to be carcinogenic. If you do take any of the medications listed, it might be important to have a discussion with your doctor regarding your need for them.

The information provided here is for reference only and is certainly not a "prescription" for you. The information is to make you aware so that you can be a proactive consumer and patient, armed with knowledge and nutritional insight.

1) Folic Acid

We looked extensively at the difference between folic acid and folate (methylfolate) in the last chapter. Let's briefly review what we read. We determined that folate is a wonderful vitamin for our health and for growing fetuses, and it helps to ward off cancer. Folic acid, on the other hand, is the synthetic, man-made version of the vitamin and is potentially dangerous to our health. The health dangers come from regularly taken high doses and/or if someone has a common gene mutation called MTHFR. A person with MTHFR cannot convert the synthetic form to the bio-available, absorbable form, so the folic acid builds up in the body, rising to potentially toxic levels.

A 2014 article written for *Alliance for Natural Health* reviewed studies regarding folic acid supplementation. The author points out that the studies finding a relationship between folic acid and cancer all found that association with synthetic folic acid, not with natural folate. It was determined that unmetabolized folic acid (UMFA) is an emerging risk for cancer. One of the cancers under scrutiny is breast cancer. Mammary tumors were increased with higher amounts of folic acid supplementation. Other cancers linked to high folic acid levels are those of the colon, lung, and prostate.

When folate intakes are from food, researchers found a more consistent and stronger picture of cancer-protective effects. Folate from food also had none of the apparent risks associated with synthetic folic acid.

So the bottom line is that if you are wanting to increase your folate levels, do so either with food or with a methylfolate supplement. (Some experts also suggest that a folinic acid supplement, derived from food and not synthetic, may be as helpful as methylfolate.) Pregnant women are often advised to increase folate to prevent neural tube defects in their babies. They should look for supplements or prenatal vitamins that contain folate not folic acid. Also, for anyone taking a daily multivitamin, it would be wise to look for a brand that contains methylfolate. Be aware that most drug store brands do contain folic acid, so you might need to search online for some that fit the bill. You can also find multivitamins that do not contain any folic acid or folate.

2) Vitamin B12 (as Cyanocobalamin)

Vitamin B12 works along with folate in the production of red blood cells. It's involved in the production of the myelin sheath which surrounds our nerves, allowing for smooth neurologic function. Vitamin B12 also aids in the formation of DNA.

However, just like folic acid, the synthetic form of B12 can be toxic to us. That synthetic form is cyanocobalamin. Again, we discussed the difference between methylcobalamin (the preferred and natural form of B12) and cyanocobalamin in the last chapter. Please reference that section for more in depth information.

Like high folic acid levels, high vitamin B12 levels can be linked with cancer. And as with folic acid, some people are not able to convert synthetic vitamin B12 to its usable form methylcobalamin. This results in high serum levels that can become toxic.

Natural News explains, "By taking low-quality cyanobalamin, you're actually stealing methyl groups from your body and making it do more work at the biochemical level. This uses up substances such as glutathione that are often in short supply anyway, potentially worsening your overall health situation rather than helping it. This is one of the reasons why low-grade vitamins may actually be worse for your body than taking nothing at all." Remember, glutathione is the "master antioxidant." We need it to prevent cancer. We don't want to do anything to drain its supply.

High levels of B12 have been found in the blood of many cancer patients. It's not clear whether the B12 is causative or if the body cannot clear B12 once cancer has infiltrated it, especially when the liver is involved. Even so, it would do consumers well to just avoid synthetic vitamin B12 and opt for methylcobalamin. Look for this form in your multivitamins. Throw away any that contain synthetic forms.

3) Vitamin E

This is a warning especially for men who may currently be supplementing or thinking of supplementing with stand-alone vitamin E. Advice given a decade ago has changed. Doctors used to suggest taking extra vitamin E due to its help with cardiovascular disease. Vitamin E is an antioxidant and was thought to help prevent heart attacks and ischemic strokes. However, more recent findings do not demonstrate that it prevents heart disease and instead show a strong correlation between vitamin E supplementation and the development of prostate cancer.

A large study called "SELECT" (Selenium and Vitamin E Cancer Prevention Trial) involved over 35,000 men selected between the years 2001 and 2004 and studied for five years. The study participants were randomly divided into four groups and given one of four supplements: selenium, vitamin E, both selenium and vitamin E, or a placebo. After following up with the participants again in 2011, the men who had taken vitamin E alone had a 17% increased risk of developing prostate cancer as opposed to the other groups. Those men had been given daily doses of 400 IU per day of a synthetic form of vitamin E, dl-alpha tocopheryl acetate.

Are you noticing a trend here? Another **synthetic** vitamin appears to be causing problems. Among those who've scrutinized the study, some believe it was the form of vitamin E that was problematic. An article in *Nutrition Science News* states that the body cannot metabolize synthetic vitamin E the way it does with natural forms. The author writes, "Researchers have found that natural vitamin E assimilates far better than synthetic versions. Specific binding and transport proteins produced in the liver select the natural d-alpha form of vitamin E and largely ignore all other forms." So basically, our livers can't process synthetic forms as easily. No one should be taking synthetic versions. Period.

Non-synthetic forms of vitamin E are labeled as d-alpha tocopherol, d-alpha tocopheryl acetate, or d-alpha tocopheryl succinate. The synthetic forms instead begin with a dl- prefix.

Like all vitamins, we do need vitamin E in the right forms and in the right quantities. We can get it from foods like almonds, seeds, leafy greens, avocado, broccoli, olives and olive oil, sweet potatoes, or papaya. Also, the amount in multivitamins is enough to cover our bases without being too much. Only 200 IU or less per day is currently recommended to avoid taking too large a dose. Also, as mentioned, the best form of vitamin E is mixed tocopherols or, more accurately, those that begin with the d-alpha prefixes. Check your multivitamins and look for those forms of vitamin E. And remember, you really do not need a stand-alone supplement of this vitamin.

4) Beta-Carotene

The concern with this supplement is again the synthetic form. The concern also has more to do with people who smoke or were smokers in regard to lung cancer. We'll get into the studies in just a moment, but please note that, once again, synthetic forms of vitamins have proven time and time again to be problematic.

Beta-carotene found in foods or in food-based vitamins is a wonderfully healthy addition to the diet. It is a substance from plants that the body converts into vitamin A. It acts as an antioxidant and immune booster. It is found in orange-yellow vegetables and dark leafy greens.

Synthetic beta-carotene, however, is not as easily converted. And like other synthetic vitamins we've looked at, toxic levels can build up and cause issues.

Synthetic beta-carotene consists of only one molecule called all trans beta-carotene. (Natural beta-carotene found in food is made of two molecules: all trans beta-carotene plus 9-cis beta-carotene.) Synthetic beta-carotene is manufactured from benzene extracted from acetylene gas. Benzene is a natural constituent of crude oil. Not only do these substances have no nutritional value, benzene is considered to be a carcinogen or cancer-causing substance.

In a study, published in 1994 in the *New England Journal of Medicine*, male smokers who took beta-carotene supplements (20 mg/day) had an 18% higher risk of lung cancer over five to eight years compared with male smokers who did not take the supplements. They also had an 8% higher risk of mortality. The finding "raised the possibility" that beta-carotene supplements are harmful to smokers. The study was first conducted because researchers believed, prior to the study, that beta-carotene showed promising benefits for health, and they hoped to help smokers prevent cancer. Surprisingly, the study found just the opposite.

I would not be overly concerned if you see beta-carotene in your multivitamin, especially if it's from a reputable source. However, there are no reasons to supplement with a stand-alone beta-carotene. As always, it would be best to get most of your beta-carotene and vitamin A from food sources.

5) Some Oral Contraceptives

If you're taking hormonal birth control or have taken it in the past, please do not worry. Remember, the information we're providing is just to give you facts regarding some studies and some trends doctors have noted. However, hormonal birth control pills or Oral Contraceptives (OCs) are most likely safe for most women. Newer, lower dose estrogen pills have proven to be much less likely to cause cancer. Some OCs are even protective *against* some forms of cancer. Nonetheless, we'll look at historical connections with OCs and cancer, and we'll mention the populations of women for whom OCs might be problematic.

First some **good news**. Combination OCs, meaning that they contain estrogen and progesterone, have been found to decrease the risk for endometrial and ovarian cancers. Even better, the anticancer effects last for up to 25 years after stopping the pill! One hypothesis is that protection is achieved by blocking ovulation. When women are on the pill, they don't ovulate. Thus the body is not exposed to the hormonal fluctuations of each monthly cycle. Scientists propose that a major source of the protection from OCs is because they significantly reduce cell proliferation in the fallopian tubes and in ovarian cysts, two likely cells of origin for ovarian cancer. As for endometrial (or uterine) cancer, OCs prevent a thickening of the uterine wall each month. The thickening and subsequent sloughing off of tissue that occurs naturally without OCs, sometimes causes cellular changes in the uterus. This can lead to the development of abnormal, precancerous cells that proliferate and then eventually become malignant.

It is interesting to note that OCs also seem to reduce the risk for colon cancer in some studies. A study found in the journal *Epidemiology* found that women who had a history of OC use had a 36% reduced risk of developing colorectal cancer. The researchers stated, "These findings are consistent with the descriptive epidemiology of colorectal cancer, the bile acid hypothesis, and experimental findings on estrogen receptors and the colorectal cancer pathway." Estrogen in the pill is thought to reduce the risk of colon cancer by decreasing bile acids that have been linked to colon cancer.

Here's the **bad news**. The use of OCs is associated with an increased risk of breast cancer. However, the amount of synthetic hormones in the pill are typically the determining factor on how likely a women is to develop the disease. High-dose estrogen OCs more than double the risk of developing breast cancer. Progestin-only OCs also double the risk. Tri-phasic OCs triple the risk. But, low-dose estrogen pills do NOT increase the risk for breast cancer. These findings were illustrated in a 2014 study in the journal *Cancer Research*.

If you are considering taking OCs or currently are, it appears that low-dose estrogen pills are the way to go. Examples of this include Norgestimate, Norethindrone acetate, and Levonorgestrel (the names may be different depending on brand and/or generic name). If you have a family history of breast cancer, or if you carry the BRCA1 or BRCA2 gene mutation, you should not take OCs. Likewise women over 40 have a slightly increased rate of developing breast cancer when taking OCs (however, some research points out that the risk really doesn't increase until closer to age 50).

6) Postmenopausal Hormone Replacement Therapy

After menopause, a woman's ovaries stop producing hormones, namely estrogen and progesterone, in the amount they used to. This can result in symptoms like hot flashes, vaginal dryness, low libido, irritability, and depression. Osteoporosis is also much more likely to occur during the menopausal years.

To combat the unwanted symptoms of menopause, women may turn to Hormone Replacement Therapy (HRT), otherwise known as Hormone Therapy (HT). This is traditionally a combination of estrogen and progesterone (or synthetic progestin). This therapy is NOT Bio-identical Hormone Replacement Therapy (BHRT), which is supposedly derived from natural sources and arguably has fewer side effects. However, BHRT hasn't been studied to the same degree and doesn't have the same approval standards. The problem with traditional HRT has been the connection between it and cancer, namely breast cancer.

The Women's Health Initiative Study, which began in the 1990s, looked at over 160,000 postmenopausal women. Clinical trials were developed to assess the use of HRT. In 2002, the study stopped giving women combination HRT because of the untoward side effects that developed. It showed that women were at an increased risk not only for cardiovascular disease but also for breast cancer.

Despite the risks, women may still benefit from HRT in the right doses. Women who experienced an early menopause, who do not have family or personal history of breast cancer, who do not smoke, and who have debilitating symptoms of menopause may be candidates. There are different forms of HRT, so work with your doctor to determine which might be best for you. It appears that taking HRT for the shortest duration possible may also help lessen the chance of developing cancer or other disease.

Some traditional doctors and many naturopathic doctors recommend BHRT instead. To date, there have been no correlations between BHRT and cancer. Whereas traditional HRT uses synthetic hormones, BHRT is said to use exact structural replicas of the hormones that are naturally produced by the body. Another added benefit of BHRT is that each dose is tailored specifically for a woman's needs, not simply what doses the pharmaceutical company offers. So, if you are a woman in peri-menopause or menopause and are experiencing symptoms, you might also want to find a provider who specializes in BHRT. As a consumer, you must do your research to find the treatment pathway that works best for you with the least amount of side effects and least amount of risk.

7) Anabolic Steroids

So you're probably thinking you can just tune out this section because, certainly, if you're not a body-builder, you needn't worry. Well, the reality is, sometimes health practitioners prescribe anabolic steroids for other reasons. Someone you know may actually be taking these for other reasons, so it's good to know what anabolic steroids are all about and why folks may take them.

Anabolic steroids are synthetic variations of the male sex hormone testosterone. The proper term for these compounds is *anabolic-androgenic steroids*. "Anabolic" refers to muscle building, and "androgenic" refers to increased male sex characteristics. Intense weight-lifters and body-builders, men and women alike, may turn to anabolic steroids to improve physical performance or to give them a competitive advantage. They are purported to increase lean body mass, strength, and aggressiveness.

Health care providers can prescribe anabolic steroids to treat hormonal issues, such as delayed puberty. These steroids can also treat diseases that cause muscle loss, such as cancer and AIDS. (*Be aware that these are NOT *corticosteroids* that are commonly used by doctors to treat various levels of inflammation.) So, although not commonly prescribed, anabolic steroids can be and are used by doctors to treat some patients as well. Typically though, the amount prescribed by doctors is much lower than the amount abused by body-builders.

A major issue is that often when body-builders take anabolic steroids, they do so without a prescription and in massive doses. This is toxic to their overall health, not to mention illegal.

Some side effects of long-term anabolic steroid use are mental health issues (like paranoia and irritability), kidney and liver problems, enlarged heart, elevated blood pressure, and stroke. For men, gynecomastia, shrinking testes, decreased sperm count, and baldness may occur. For women taking anabolic steroids, they may experience loss of period, a deepened voice, growth of facial and body hair. If teens take these steroids, they may also have stunted growth or height.

Those are some pretty nasty effects, but probably the most worrisome is the potential for cancer. Men who have taken anabolic steroids are at an increased risk for prostate cancer. Steroid abuse is also linked with tumors of the liver, probably because the liver must process all medications and toxins that enter the body.

If your doctor treats you or a loved one with anabolic steroids, the benefits probably outweigh the risks. However, if you know someone taking anabolic steroids for muscle growth and fitness purposes, be aware that the damage created may be irreversible. Also, if someone has a personal or family history of prostate cancer, liver disease or failure, or liver cancer, anabolic steroids should absolutely be avoided.

8) Human Growth Hormone

Human growth hormone (HGH) is naturally produced in the pituitary gland. Our bodies release HGH to promote growth in children and adolescents. HGH is also responsible for cell growth and regeneration, and it helps with muscle mass and bone density. After we stop growing, HGH levels plummet.

Because of its effects on muscle growth, it is another substance that body-builders sometimes turn to. HGH seems to be the modern-day, more "acceptable," and supposedly safer version of steroids. Like anabolic steroids, HGH can also be prescribed by physicians to treat various health-related issues. And also like anabolic steroids, use of HGH can be abused.

First off, we need natural HGH to develop and grow as children. Doctors may also prescribe extra injections of HGH to children whose growth has stalled or been delayed due to small gestational size, kidney disease, or other genetic conditions. In adults, HGH may be used to treat muscle wasting, short bowel syndrome, or HGH deficiency due to pituitary tumors.

In adult bodies, naturally produced HGH is needed for strong bones and muscles, maintaining cardiovascular health, for good moods, and adequate sleep. Deficiencies of HGH are linked with depression, sexual dysfunction, memory loss, increased triglycerides, insulin resistance, osteoporosis, fatigue, and weight gain. So, we do need an adequate amount to function optimally.

However, the off-label uses of HGH are of true concern. Some tout that supplemental HGH is an anti-aging agent. It is purported to increase muscle mass, increase energy, improve the appearance of skin and hair, reduce joint and muscle pain, etc. But taking HGH, especially in high doses, can be problematic. If taken in excess, HGH can abnormally increase bones and muscles. This is called acromegaly. Overuse of HGH can also lead to cardiac conditions like irregular heartbeats and an enlarged heart. Kidney damage has also been associated with its use.

There is not a definitive link between HGH and cancer, but some studies have shown some correspondence. A 2004 article in the journal *Drug Safety* pointed some causation of cancer to HGH. It stated that since HGH is anabolic, it allows for cell proliferation (normal or cancerous cells). It is also anti-apoptotic (preventing cancer cell death) because it turns into insulin-like growth factor (IGF-1) in the liver. We know that there is an association between high IGF-1 and cancer. The article cited a study follow-up of pituitary HGH recipients that suggested an increase in colorectal cancer. In addition, follow-up of oncology patients suggested an increase in second cancers in those who also received HGH therapy. On the other hand, children given HGH to stimulate growth did not appear to have risk for cancer later in life.

So, unless your doctor prescribes HGH for you, it is best to increase HGH naturally, without HGH supplements or drugs. To naturally boost

HGH, one can do several things. Vigorous exercise for at least 10 minutes boosts levels. Think HIIT exercises (High Intensity Interval Training). Supplementing with certain amino acids may also help. L-glutamine and l-arginine are reported to boost HGH. Vitamin C is also thought to increase natural levels of HGH. Intermittent fasting (which we'll discuss in Chapter 7) can also do the trick. Working out in a fasted state is especially useful in upping HGH levels. One study even concluded that watching a funny movie boosts HGH by 27%. Laughter just may be the best medicine!

9) Long-Term Use of Corticosteroids

Corticosteroids are used by doctors to treat various inflammatory conditions. They may also be referred to as glucocorticoids, which are a sub category. (These are NOT the anabolic steroids mentioned previously.) They may go by the names prednisone, hydrocortisone, cortisone, dexamethasone, or methylprednisolone to name a few. Note, they usually end in an -one suffix.

Use of corticosteroids ranges anywhere from the treatment of hives to much more critical conditions like preventing organ failure from transplants. You may hear of people being prescribed these steroids for allergic reactions, arthritis, colitis, bronchitis, asthma, lupus, or other autoimmune conditions.

These steroids absolutely have a place in modern medicine and can be life saving. If your doctor prescribes steroids, you will most likely benefit from taking them. The following information that will be presented is only to warn you of some long-term consequences of steroid use so that you and your doctor can have a conversation. You should never go off of these steroids without first consulting your doctor. There is a weaning approach that is typically necessary to avoid undue side effects. You must taper off taking these before you stop completely.

Side effects of long-term or heavy-dose corticosteroids are fluid retention, weight gain, puffy face, high blood pressure, loss of potassium, headache, mood swings, muscle weakness, muscle wasting, thinning and bruising of the skin, slow wound healing, glaucoma, cataracts, ulcers in the mouth or digestive tract, osteoporosis, and diabetes. Sounds pretty terrible, right? They can be.

Corticosteroids help to reduce inflammation by suppressing the immune system. However, this can lead to infections, illness, and even cancer. Research from a 2004 Danish study showed a connection between steroid use and skin malignancies (basal cell and squamous cell) and non-Hodgkins lymphoma. This association was with people that had 10-15 or more steroid prescriptions filled over a seven-year period. A separate study published in 2005 did NOT find the same connection between steroid use and lymphoma. So, it appears further research needs to be completed.

Corticosteroids are actually sometimes used in the treatment of cancer. They may work as an adjuvant with chemotherapy and to decrease inflammation associated with cancer treatments.

So, these types of steroids are not a "cut and dry" yes or no. They may be very helpful, and they may cause awful side effects. Again, if you need them, they may be wonderfully effective. Just be aware that long-term use can have potentially dangerous side effects. Shorter-term use, if possible, is best for your body. If you or a loved one are taking corticosteroids, be extra careful to look for any negative side effects so that you can report them to your doctor. You and your doctor must work together on your health plan.

10) Excessive Use of Antibiotics

The overuse of antibiotics in our society is no secret. Recently, we've heard warnings against asking your doctor for antibiotics when they are not needed. We've also heard of doctors over-prescribing them. The problem is that overuse leads to resistant strains of bacteria. Essentially, less harmful bacteria can be wiped out leaving harmful, more virulent, bacteria behind. Antibiotic resistance occurs when bacteria change in some way that reduces or eliminates the effectiveness of drugs, chemicals, or other agents designed to cure or prevent infections. The bacteria survive and continue to multiply causing more harm. Then, the "go-to" antibiotics no longer work, and doctors must turn to last-resort antibiotics to treat infections. And sadly, in rare occurrences, people may develop especially resistant strains of bacteria that cannot be treated at all without hospitalization and isolation.

Antibiotics can and should only be used to treat bacterial infections. Viral infections like the common cold and even the flu do not respond to antibiotics. Also, sometimes people stop taking their antibiotics when they begin to feel better. This is also a big "no-no." If treatment stops too soon, some bacteria may persist and re-infect.

We also know that too many antibiotics can wipe out the body's good bacteria, allowing for an overgrowth of yeast or candida. Many women have been reported to develop yeast infections after a dose or two of antibiotics. Unfortunately, yeast isn't always so obvious in the body and can linger for years untreated. Yeast can cause things like headaches, dizziness, infections, brain fog, joint pain, etc. A Rome-based oncologist, Dr. Tullio Simoncini, says that cancer is actually a fungus, an advanced form of candida overgrowth. It's an interesting theory to say the least. If nothing else, an overgrowth of yeast is yet another unpleasant and unwanted side effect to taking antibiotics.

A traditional study published in the *Journal of the American Medical Association* (JAMA) reveals that any use of antibiotics potentially increases the risk of breast cancer in women. The specific data for this study states that women who took only 1 to 25 antibiotics over a 17-year period had a one and a half times higher risk of breast cancer as compared to women who took no antibiotics. The study's author was quick to point out that this doesn't mean antibiotics caused the cancer, only that there is a correlation between the two.

Dr. Roberta Nessa, an epidemiologist from the University of Pittsburgh, co-authored an editorial that accompanied this study. She says, "What we thought was perhaps the more likely explanation is that the antibiotics themselves are not what's the problem here, but in fact they're marking the reason why women take antibiotics and that is infection. Chronic infection causes chronic inflammation and we know that inflammation causes a series of different cancers."

So, what comes first? The chicken or the egg? Can antibiotics cause cancer or do chronic infections that require antibiotics cause it? The take away message is this ... Try to find the root cause of infections to avoid them from occurring. Follow an overall healthy diet and lifestyle, limiting inflammatory foods and getting adequate exercise and sleep. Limit antibiotic use when possible because, regardless if they cause cancer, they have unwanted side effects when used in abundance. Only take antibiotics when they are absolutely needed.

Final Thoughts on Supplements & Meds to Limit or Avoid

As we age, we will probably inevitably be prescribed some medications. Some will be necessary to treat various conditions like high blood pressure, high cholesterol, heart disease, or loss of cognitive function. Others might be optional like antidepressants. Some medications could be prescribed to treat the side effects of other medications. Examples would be taking stool softeners or laxatives because pain medications have caused constipation, or taking Ativan to reduce the nausea involved with chemo. Taking an abundance of medications is called "polypharmacy," and it's become a real problem in our population. This practice increases the risk for adverse drug reactions, falls, hospitalization, institutionalization, mortality, and other detrimental health outcomes.

You may not be able to avoid taking some or all medications, but you can read the labels. Always, always look for side effects and potential interactions with other medications. Weigh the options. Do you absolutely need the medication? Can the problem be fixed through diet or lifestyle? Do the benefits of taking the drug outweigh the risks? What exactly are the side effects that could occur so you can be on the lookout? Are there studies that have been done on the medication and what are the findings? Be proactive and a prudent consumer.

Even if you are not on medications, you'll likely take some supplements ... as you should! We discussed many beneficial supplements in the last chapter. In this chapter, we looked at some that are not as savory. Just as with medication, be aware of what you're putting into your body. Do not just take any old multivitamin. Look for those without synthetic vitamins, as we discussed. Pay for a well-rounded, reputable brand that contains methylated versions especially of B12 and folate. Also, don't take any stand-alone supplements that you're unsure of or feel you do not need. Don't take something just because your next door neighbor does or because you heard about it on TV. Do your research and understand the benefits of supplements versus the risks. Be sure the supplements you take are for nourishment, for immunity, and overall health, not because they are touted as weight-loss miracles or get-ripped-quick gimmicks.

Medications and supplements can do great things, but sometimes they can hurt us if taken in the wrong doses, taken haphazardly, or taken for too long. You are in charge of your body. Your doctor may guide you, but always know you have a choice in what you put in your body. Take care of yourself on all levels and be your own strongest advocate. Listen to your intuition, but also do your research.

---

* Anticancer Action *

Go through your current collection of supplements and vitamins. Throw out your multivitamin if it contains folic acid or cyanocobalamin (synthetic B12). Get rid of any supplements that are expired. And if you can't remember why you bought some, toss those, too.

Chapter 6: Environmental Toxins to Avoid

We all know pollution is bad for us. If you're like me, when you picture "pollution," you probably think of thick, gray smoke-filled air. When I was a little girl in the 1970s, my grandparents lived near a coke plant. Coke is a by-product of coal. In the summers, before my sister and I were allowed to play on their big front porch, my mother and grandmother had to wipe down all the soot and dirt that covered the furniture and walls. Of course, that sort of pollution is obvious, and obviously harmful. However, there are forms of "pollution" and toxins all around us. Some may be in household products you use every day. Some may be in cleaners. Others may be in beauty products. Other forms of pollution cannot even be seen by the naked eye, like radiation. In this chapter, we'll cover a few of the major environmental toxins. Of course, since we live in a modern world, it's impossible to avoid them all. However, there are ways to limit your exposure, and you can learn to be a savvy consumer as well.

1) Dry Cleaning

You have that beautiful dress or great suit that you only wear once in a while on special occasions, but it's "dry clean only." You want to keep it looking good, so you take it to the dry cleaners then stash it away in your closet until next time. The problem is, you may be bringing toxic chemicals into your home. Did you know that you're supposed to remove the dry cleaning bag as soon as you pick up your clothing? Leaving your clothes in the bags might trap humidity or make it hard to lose any residual odor from the chemicals.

What chemicals are we talking about? Professional cleaning processes use a liquid solvent to dissolve stains on garments. This typically involves a chemical known as perc that, while highly effective at getting scuff marks out of clothing, is also a known health and environmental hazard. Perc is perchloroethylene, also known as tetrachloroethylene or PCE. In 2012, the EPA classified perc as a "likely human carcinogen," meaning that prolonged exposure to the chemical has been linked to an increased risk of cancer.

In the EPA's 2012 press release on the subject, the agency warned: "Studies of dry cleaning workers exposed to tetrachloroethylene have shown associations between exposure and several types of cancer, specifically bladder cancer, non-Hodgkin lymphoma and multiple myeloma." The EPA is trying to phase out the use of perc by dry cleaners by 2020.

Wearing dry cleaned fabrics is only mildly toxic. Dry cleaning's detriments have more to do with breathing in the pollutants through the air and also though contaminated soils. Living near a dry cleaner that uses perc puts one at greater risk for developing cancer. A 2009 study in the *Journal of Environmental and Public Health* found that those living close to a dry cleaning facility increased the risk of developing kidney cancer. If dry cleaners use proper ventilation, that risk decreases.

It may be expensive for dry cleaners to replace the use of perc with something more sustainable which is one reason it hasn't been phased out completely. GreenEarth is one alternative to perc which uses water-based cleaners, carbon dioxide, and other Earth-friendly chemicals.

What can you do? Surprisingly, many dry clean only fabrics can be hand-washed and laid flat to dry. If you must use dry cleaning, you can limit how often. Ask your local dry cleaners if they use perc and, if so, ask what sort of ventilation they use. Encourage the use of eco-friendly chemicals, and only use dry cleaners that seek out those systems.

2) Harmful Beauty Product Ingredients

We all use beauty products. They are not just make-up. These include everything from shampoo to lotions to deodorant. There are certain ingredients in some of these products that are thought to be carcinogenic or potentially toxic in large doses.

One problem with personal care products is that they typically go directly onto skin. This allows them to be almost directly absorbed into our bloodstream, then into the lymphatic system and internal organs.

Another problem is that many ingredients have not been tested for safety. According to the Environmental Working Group, the government cannot mandate safety standards for beauty products. Only 11% of the over 10,000 ingredients used in cosmetics have been assessed for safety. The remaining ingredients are used in over 90% of beauty products. It's frightening to not know if what we're putting on our bodies is safe.

The National Institute of Occupational Safety and Health reported that there are nearly 900 toxic chemicals used in cosmetics. According to a 2000 press release from the Cancer Coalition, "Cancer and health risk experts recently concluded reviews that indicate mainstream cosmetics and personal hygiene products pose the highest cancer risk exposures to the general public, even higher than smoking."

There are way too many potentially hazardous substances to mention them all, however, there are a few that tend to be used in many beauty products. Here are some common ones:

* Sodium laureth sulfate (SLS)
* Parabens
* Phthalates
* Paraffin
* Petrolatum
* Hydroquinone
* Antibacterials / Triclosans
* Mercury
* Lead

* Formaldehyde
* Nano particles
* 1,4-Dioxane / Polyethylene glycols
* BHA and BHT
* DEA
* Siloxanes
* Musks / Fragrances
* Mineral oil

One other substance to mention is **talcum powder** or baby powder. There has not been a causation established, however several lawsuits have alleged that decades-long use of the product has contributed to ovarian cancer in thousands of women. These women suggest that talcum powder caused ovarian cancer because the powder particles (applied to the genital area or on sanitary napkins, diaphragms, or condoms) traveled through the vagina, uterus, and fallopian tubes to the ovary. Dr. Clarice Weinberg, from the National Institute of Environmental Health Sciences states, "There is some literature suggesting there may be a connection between genital talcum use and ovarian cancer. It's not entirely consistent." So, if you're using talcum powder, it may be wise to keep it away from such sensitive areas. It might also be a good idea to avoid it in babies as well.

In general, when you are buying personal care items, ideally look for organic ones. Also look for those made with natural, plant-based ingredients. Oils like coconut oil or jojoba can be used to cleanse skin and/or to moisturize. Essential oils are also great for natural fragrance and antioxidant qualities. Some people swear by baking soda for washing hair, brushing teeth, and as a natural deodorant.

Again, the take away message is to read labels. Products with the most ingredients, especially ingredients you cannot pronounce or have never heard of, probably contain the most harmful constituents. Organic and naturally derived products will most likely cost a bit more, but remember that anything you put on your skin gets absorbed into your body.

3) Fluoride

You might be thinking right now that this is crazy. How could fluoride be a problem? Isn't it in most toothpastes and drinking water? Yes, my friends, it is, and if some of the research is true, fluoride may also be a really scary substance.

In the early 1900s, a dentist named Dr. Frederick McKay first discovered that in Colorado Springs, CO, the children of the town had stained brown teeth. After examination, he discovered that although the teeth were mottled, they were resistant to dental cavities. After much exploration and research into the water systems of other towns seeing the same issue, Dr. McKay found that high levels of fluoride in the water caused this occurrence. With the help of scientists, they were able to decipher which level of fluoride would be enough to prevent cavities without also staining the teeth. Hence, government-led mandates on fluoridated water began.

Not all states mandate fluoridated water. And in those that do, there is criticism. As we'll see, fluoride is not without controversy.

The most popular and highly recommended water filtration system today is "reverse osmosis." If you use a reverse osmosis filter, the fluoride will be removed. Likewise, most bottled waters do not contain fluoride. This is not by accident.

Although fluoride has been found to help with dental cavities, it is also considered a neurotoxin, especially in high doses. A 2012 meta-analysis of studies cited in *Environmental Health Perspectives* found an adverse effect of high fluoride exposure on children's neurodevelopment. In 2012, Harvard researchers reported that 26 of the 27 studies they reviewed found that childhood IQ decreased with increased fluoride concentrations.

The problem, especially in regard to young children, is that not only might they get fluoride through drinking water, but they may also ingest way too much through toothpaste. Children often swallow toothpaste. Have you even noticed the warning labels on fluoride toothpaste? It reads, "Keep out of reach of children under 6 years of age. If more than used for brushing is accidentally swallowed, seek professional help or contact a poison control center immediately." There is a reason you're supposed to spit out the toothpaste and froth that forms.

A 2014 article in *The Scientific World Journal* looked at fluoride with a critical eye. The authors write,

> *[We] conclude that available evidence suggests that fluoride has a potential to cause major adverse human health problems, while having only a modest dental caries prevention effect. As part of efforts to reduce hazardous fluoride ingestion, the practice of artificial water fluoridation should be reconsidered globally, while industrial safety measures need to be tightened in order to reduce unethical discharge of fluoride compounds into the environment. Public health approaches for global dental caries reduction that do not involve systemic ingestion of fluoride are urgently needed.*

In their scientific review, they note that fluoride's benefits to teeth occur when applied topically such that it doesn't need to be ingested. In addition, adequate calcium and magnesium are needed in teeth enamel for fluoride to be effective. So, people need to have adequate mineral content to start with. This also suggests that these minerals are much more important to human health, especially in regard to teeth and bones. Fluoride is NOT needed internally in our bodies. It is not an essential nutrient, and is not required for any body system functioning. It is only an adjuvant to minerals when applied to the teeth.

There are some published connections with fluoride and cancer. None of these have shown absolute causation, and some scientists argue that the studies are weak. Many of the studies are retrospective, meaning that researchers examined the history of increased fluoridation with increasing cancer rates. However, we'll look at some possible links between fluoride and cancer.

Population-based studies suggest that chronic fluoride ingestion is a possible cause of bladder and uterine cancer. It's important to note that those particular findings were from the 1970s and likely were in regard to very high levels of fluoride.

More modern research shows there may be a link with osteosarcoma (a type of bone cancer). A small study in 2012 published in the *South Asian Journal of Cancer* determined a link between osteosarcoma patients and high fluoride levels when compared to healthy volunteers. Another study in 2006 found that, in males under age 20 with osteosarcoma, higher levels of fluoride exposure were associated with the disease. The researchers did not find that same connection with females.

However, fluoride tends to accumulate in calcified tissue and in bone. So, just because fluoride was found in bone from patients with osteosarcoma does not mean that this caused the disease. A 2011 study showed no connection between fluoride and osteosarcoma. So the jury is still out.

Fluoride does also interfere with thyroid function. It has not been associated with thyroid cancer, however. Historically, fluoride was used to treat hyperthyroidism and Graves disease because it blocked thyroid functioning, essentially shutting off a too speedy thyroid. People who have hypothyroidism or Hashimotos should be wary of getting too much fluoride.

High levels of fluoride also contribute to fluorosis. As mentioned, fluoride can accumulate in the body. This is often seen in teeth and bones. Dental fluorosis (or mottled enamel) is an extremely common disorder, characterized by hypo-mineralization of tooth enamel caused by ingestion of excessive fluoride during enamel formation. Skeletal fluorosis is a bone disease caused by excessive accumulation of fluoride in the bones. In advanced cases, skeletal fluorosis causes pain and damage to bones and joints.

So, we can see that fluoride in high levels is not good for us. So what can we do? First, don't panic. Safety measures have been set in place by most municipalities to ensure that drinking water does not contain too much fluoride. The EPA's maximum contaminant level for fluoride in drinking water was 4 mg/L, but a so-called secondary level of 2 mg/L was set to protect against cosmetic dental effects linked to excess fluoride consumption. According to the most recent data, about 1.4 million people have water with 2 mg/L of fluoride. If your drinking water comes from a public source, you can find out about the levels of fluoride by contacting your local community water system.

If you're at all worried about drinking water, you can purchase a reverse osmosis water system. These systems remove other harmful chemicals as well. Most bottled waters and distilled waters do not contain fluoride.

If you have children, do not let them use fluoride toothpaste until they can adequately spit out the toothpaste and foam. "Training toothpastes" that do not contain fluoride are available at most drug stores.

You can reduce your consumption of processed beverages like sodas, juices, or sports drinks. These likely use fluoridated water as an ingredient. Some wines, both white and red, contain fluoride. This is because the grapes are sprayed with a pesticide containing fluoride. To avoid this, look for organic wines. This also applies to grapes and raisins.

Some research has found that cooking with Teflon-coated pans (i.e., stick-free pans) can significantly increase the fluoride content of food. If you have Teflon pans, therefore, consider switching to stainless steel.

Another surprising source of fluoride is in chicken nuggets, fingers, or patties. Mechanical deboning processes actually pulverize bone, leaving fragments behind which are incorporated into the nuggets. Chickens tend to have higher levels of fluoride in their bones than any other animal.

Teas, especially bottled and instant varieties, contain fluoride. The tea plant accumulates high levels of fluoride. However, younger leaves tend to have less, so drinking "white" tea appears to be superior in this regard. Overall, teas contain antioxidants which balance out the fluoride. So, your average teas are probably quite beneficial. Just try to avoid the bottled and instant teas since they contain much fewer levels of antioxidants.

Although it appears fluoride toothpaste is fine, if not ingested, newer non-fluoride approaches are becoming popular. Probiotics, xylitol, and biofilms also show increasing promise in cavity prevention with a strong safety profile in relation to human health.

4) Non-stick Cookware

Non-stick cookware is often coated with polytetrafluoroethylene (PTFE), otherwise known as the brand name Teflon. It creates a frictionless texture to pots and pans. Perfluorooctanoic acid (PFOA), also known as C8, is another man-made chemical. It is used in the process of making Teflon.

The International Agency for Research on Cancer has determined that PFOA is "possibly carcinogenic to humans" based on limited evidence in humans that it can cause testicular and kidney cancer. The EPA stated that there is "suggestive evidence of carcinogenicity, but not sufficient to assess human carcinogenic potential."

Manufacturers state that while PFOA is used in making Teflon, it is not present (or is present in extremely small amounts) in Teflon-coated products. However, the Environmental Working Group disagrees. They say toxic fumes from the Teflon chemical released from pots and pans at high temperatures may kill pet birds and cause people to develop flu-like symptoms (called "Teflon Flu"). Also, chemicals from this family are associated with smaller birth weight and size in newborn babies, elevated cholesterol, abnormal thyroid hormone levels, liver inflammation, and weakened immune defense against disease.

The EWG recommends using stainless steel or cast iron cookware. They also recommend never preheating non-stick cookware at high heat because empty pans can rapidly reach high temperatures. Heat at the lowest temperature possible to cook your food safely. Use an exhaust fan in the kitchen when cooking with non-stick cookware.

5) Volatile Organic Compounds

Volatile Organic Compounds, or VOCs for short, can include highly toxic chemicals such as formaldehyde and acetaldehyde, benzene, toluene, perchloroethylene, and more. These can be released from new carpeting in your home or in your car. In the short term, VOCs can cause eye irritation, headaches, nausea, or respiratory symptoms. However, long term exposure can increase your risk of cancer.

Besides off-gassing from carpeting and new furniture, VOCs can be released from paint and varnishes. Carpeting, its backing, and adhesives contain a plethora of chemicals. When carpeting is installed, the highest off-gassing of VOCs occurs in the first 72 hours. However, they can be emitted in smaller doses for years.

Other indoor sources of VOCs include air fresheners, glues, wood burning stoves, gasoline, flooring, car exhaust (if you have an integral garage), tobacco smoke, and office equipment like printers and copiers. As you can see, they are everywhere and in many objects.

The Centers for Disease Control (CDC) lists the following VOCs as potentially harmful: *ethylenezene, benzene, xylene, toluene, styrene, carbon tetrachloride, 1,1,1-Trichloroethane, Tetrachloroethylene, also known as perchloroethylene, Trichloroethylene, and 1,4-dichlorobenzene.* On their website, the CDC talks about each of these separately. They point out that most of these, in small doses, cause things like respiratory issues and headaches, but that in much higher doses many were carcinogenic to animals in lab studies.

Most are not associated with cancer in humans except for a few (although each has long-term neurologic and organ-related consequences with higher exposures).

* Benzene: Long-term exposure to high levels of benzene in the air can cause a particular type of leukemia called acute myelocytic leukemia. Benzene comes from burning coal and oil and from motor vehicle exhaust.

* Xylene: Studies on xylene have shown an association with cancer. Xylene is used in solvents, and in printing, rubber, and leather industries.

* **Styrene:** This is another that can cause leukemia or lymphoma as has been seen in workers making styrene-based products. Styrene is used to make some plastic products and packaging materials.

* **Carbon tetrachloride:** It potentially causes cancer and is used to make refrigeration fluid and propellants for aerosol cans. It accumulates in fatty tissues and has been found to generate liver tumors in lab animals.

* **Trichloroethylene:** This is mainly used as a solvent and is also found in adhesives and spot removers. It can leach into ground water. Studies of people exposed over long periods to high levels of trichloroethylene in drinking water found more heart defects and cancer such as leukemia.

* **Formaldehyde:** Formaldehyde is a colorless, strong-smelling gas used in making building materials and many household products. It too has been associated with cancer risk. You would find formaldehyde in things like pressed wood products, adhesives and glues, insulations, industrial disinfectants, preservatives in funeral homes, tobacco smoke, and air fresheners. The main exposure for humans is through inhalation. High exposures can increase the risk of developing nasopharyngeal cancer. Studies show this increase in workers that manufacture products with formaldehyde and in funeral embalmers. Several studies have found that embalmers, medical professionals, and industrial workers that use formaldehyde have an increased risk of leukemia, particularly myeloid leukemia.

You can protect yourself against most high-level exposures to VOCs. Buy "low VOC" paint and building supplies. Dispose of leftover paint appropriately. Most communities have systems for hazardous waste collection. Open windows and use a fan when you first get new carpeting or furniture and when working with certain paints and adhesives. Hard wood or tile flooring tend to be more eco-friendly options. However, some carpeting manufacturers sell "greener" versions made with wool or that have a "Green Label Plus" tag indicating safer standards. Also, try to stay away from air fresheners that plug in or are sprayed into the air with aerosol cans or spray bottles. These contain a multitude of VOCs and other nasty chemicals that are associated with cancer.

Flame retardants are also added to carpeting and contain VOCs as well. These flame retardants are also in furniture upholstery. And, they turn up in children's products such as car seats, changing table pads, portable crib mattresses, nap mats, pajamas, and nursing pillows. Of course, this is a safety feature to prevent children from being burned, but their skin and lungs are then exposed to these retardants. Read the labels, especially on babies and children's items, to check if they are treated with these chemicals.

6) Some Household Cleaning Products

The latest trend in household cleaning is to buy "green" cleaners: "all natural," organic, or eco-friendly products. This is because we're becoming more and more aware of the toxins being emitted into our air from traditional, chemical-laden cleaning supplies.

There are a host of unhealthy chemicals in cleaning products, but we'll take a look at a few of the worst offenders.

* **Phthalates:** These are usually hidden behind the word "fragrance." We also looked at these in the harmful beauty products section. They can be in any cleaner that is scented. They are also definitely in air fresheners. Be aware that phthalates are in vinyl shower curtains as well. Most exposure to them is through inhalation. Phthalates are known endocrine disruptors. Endocrine disruptors are chemicals that interfere with hormones. If you choose fragrance-free or, even better, organic products, you are likely to avoid phthalates.

* **Triclosan:** This chemical is often seen in hand sanitizers. It's also used in soap and detergents that are labeled "antibacterial." It can promote the growth of drug-resistant bacteria. Triclosan is considered a probable carcinogen and possible endocrine disruptor. To avoid this, use soaps that are NOT labeled antibacterial, and use hand sanitizers that are alcohol-based.

* **Quarternary Ammonium Compounds (QUATS):** These are commonly found in fabric softener liquids and sheets. They are also antimicrobial and can breed antibiotic resistant bacteria. They are associated with respiratory disorders and asthma. You can actually use plain white vinegar as a fabric softener. It does the trick and also doesn't leave behind a vinegar smell.

* **2-Butoxyethanol:** This is found in window cleaners and multi-purpose cleaners. It gives window cleaners that characteristic sweet smell.

It is a "glycol ether." According to the EPA, glycol ethers can cause pulmonary edema, and liver and kidney damage. If you're using window cleaners or similar multi-purpose cleaners, keep the area well-ventilated. Even better, use vinegar and water to clean mirrors and windows. You can also use vinegar, baking soda, and some good smelling essential oils to clean most surfaces like kitchen counters and bathroom sinks.

* **Ammonia:** This is often used in products that clean bathroom fixtures, sinks, and jewelry and is also in glass cleaners. Ammonia is a lung irritant and can lead to chronic bronchitis and asthma. Ammonia also creates a *poisonous* gas if mixed with bleach. So, be very careful never to combine the two. A cool natural alternative is vodka. It gives a superb shine, and you can have a cocktail while you clean! If you're looking for a silver / jewelry polish, try toothpaste.

* **Chlorine:** Chlorine is found in scouring powders, toilet bowl cleaners, mildew removers, laundry whiteners, and even household tap water. You can be exposed to this through skin, through inhalation, and even when consuming tap water. It can cause lung irritation and is also known to cause thyroid issues. Here again you can use vinegar to clean surfaces and even laundry. To avoid chlorine in tap water, install a filter in your kitchen and maybe even in your shower to avoid chlorine from touching the skin.

* **Sodium Hydroxide:** This is also known as lye. It is very corrosive and also a major skin irritant. If it is inhaled it can cause throat and lung irritation. This is found in oven cleaners and in drain openers. You should

have an extremely well-ventilated room when using these, and also use a mask and gloves when dealing with lye. All natural oven cleaners are baking soda scrubs. To unclog drains, first try mechanical methods like a "snake." You can also try pouring a cup of baking soda and a cup of vinegar down the drain and let it sit for 30 minutes. After the bubbles die down, run boiling or hot water down the drain to clear the debris.

You can avoid harmful chemicals by looking for alternatives to chemical disinfectants or use organic cleaning products. We mentioned vinegar and baking soda. You can also try antibacterial, antifungal tea-tree oil. Mix a few drops of tea-tree oil and a tablespoon of vinegar with water in a spray bottle for a safe, germ-killing, all-purpose cleaner. You can also add a couple of drops of lavender or eucalyptus essential oil for scent.

7) Gel Manicures

This makes me very sad because I love a gel mani! The nail color stays on a long time without chipping and looks so shiny. To be honest, I'll still occasionally get gel manicures for special events (and sometimes just because I like them), but it is certainly best to limit how often we treat ourselves to them.

The main issue with a gel manicure is that ultraviolet (UV) lights are used to dry and set the polish. Although many UV lamps that have been studied emit low-level radiation, there is no standard or regulation on the lamps. So, if you frequently get these manicures, the radiation can add up over time.

UV radiation has been associated with skin cancer and even dangerous melanoma. Before getting a gel mani, apply sunscreen to your fingers, hands, wrists, and arms. You can also purchase fingerless photo protective gloves.

Some researchers even go so far as to say you should wear sunglasses when using UV lights. It is especially problematic for workers at salons that are exposed to these lights every day. The lights are associated with the development of cataracts, macular degeneration, and even skin cancer around the eyes.

Another issues with gel manicures is that in order to take off the polish, you must soak your fingers in acetone for 15 minutes or so. Acetone essentially disintegrates the polish, making it easier to scrape off. Acetone is an irritant when inhaled. You can try removing gel polish without acetone, but it must be soaked much longer and will probably need to be scraped or filed off mechanically, which really destroys the underlying nail.

Gel polish also tends to ruin one's nails and cuticles. The polish blocks oxygen transfer through the nail, and nails can emerge discolored and thin. A person's nail can even separate from the nail bed, or turn green due to infections that were hidden by the polish.

So, taking breaks between gel manicures seems to be the best bet. This reduces UV exposure and allows the nails time to breathe in between polishes. Getting regular/standard manicures are much safer. However, the results do not last nearly as long.

8) Tanning Beds

This is another luxury for men and women alike. And this is also another form of UV radiation exposure. Typically, when people visit tanning salons, they visit them more than once in a short duration of time. Some even have regular weekly visits. Over time, this exposure to ultraviolet light adds up and become hazardous. Not only do tanning beds add to wrinkling and decreased elasticity of the skin, but they are also associated with an increased skin cancer risk.

The famous Nurse's study which followed more than 70,000 nurses over a 20 year period found an increased risk in skin cancer, especially of basal cell carcinoma, in those who used tanning beds. Interestingly, the younger the age of exposure, the more likely a person was to develop this cancer. Those under 35 with a tanning bed history had a higher incidence of skin cancer. In fact, using tanning beds before age 30 increases one's risk of developing melanoma by 75%.

The Melanoma Research Foundation states that as many as 90% of melanoma cases are directly related to UV exposure. Melanoma is considered the deadliest form of skin cancer. The World Health Organization's International Agency for Research on Cancer (IARC) classifies tanning beds and tanning lamps into its highest cancer risk category – "carcinogenic to humans," the same category as other hazardous substances such as plutonium and certain types of radium. The Melanoma Foundation also states that even occasional tanning bed use triples one's risk of developing the disease, so they advise against any use whatsoever.

Do not be misled to believe that tanning beds offer a boost of vitamin D. The fact is, most tanning beds shed UVA rays. UVB rays are needed to produce vitamin D. Supplementing with vitamin D or getting 15 minutes of natural sunlight are much safer alternatives. "Sunless" tanning is also an option for those wishing for a sun-kissed glow. Creams and lotions, especially organic, are safe and rather effective. Be careful and do your research if you decide to get a spray tan. Both lotions and spray tans use DHA (dihydroxyacetone). This is FDA approved, however inhalation of DHA is not recommended. So, if you do get a spray tan, use precautions. The FDA recommends using nose plugs, wearing goggles, wearing lip balm, wearing protective undergarments, and ensuring there is proper ventilation. All of these recommendations are designed to protect one from inhaling the mist and/or getting it on mucous membranes (like lips or genital areas).

9) Radon

Radon is a colorless, odorless gas, and it may be lurking in your home or workplace without you even knowing it. Radon can enter homes through cracks in floors, walls, or foundations, and collect indoors. It can also be released from building materials. Radon levels can be higher in homes that are well insulated, tightly sealed, and/or built on soil rich in the elements uranium, thorium, and radium. Basement and first floors typically have the highest radon levels because of their closeness to the ground.

When my husband and I bought our home, we discovered via the inspection that the house's radon levels were "through the roof." Our realtor told us they were the highest she'd ever seen. We needed to have a system installed. Radon mitigation systems work to pull radon out of the house. Systems extend a slight vacuum under the home to pull this air away from living spaces and direct it towards the outside. A fan and vent pipe are used to draw air out from under a basement, crawl space, or concrete slab, pulling the air outside.

Radon is dangerous because it is the second leading cause of lung cancer. Radon decays quickly, giving off tiny radioactive particles. When inhaled, these radioactive particles can damage the cells that line the lung.

If you are worried about the radon levels in your home, you can even purchase a "do-it-yourself" testing kit. Look for test kits online or at home centers and hardware stores, with prices ranging from about $9 to $40. You can also contact your state radon office to find out if they offer a low-cost or free test kit. If your home does contain radon, mitigation systems can be installed by professional companies. They typically range from $800 to $1500.

10) Cell Phones

There is some controversy as to whether or not cell phones actually are associated with harmful radiation and cancer. The majority of studies on cell phones and brain cancer are inconclusive. In 2011, the World Health Organization classified cell phone use as "possibly carcinogenic to humans," based on limited and inconsistent evidence from human studies, and limited evidence from studies of radio-frequency energy and cancer in rodents.

Cell phones produce radio-frequency. Radio-frequency energy is a form of electro-magnetic radiation. It is considered "non-ionizing" which is extremely low energy or energy from that of power. This is different from "ionizing" energy which is associated with things like radon and x-rays. Ionizing radiation, in high doses, IS associated with cancer.

The FDA, the CDC, the National Institute of Environmental Health Sciences, and the Federal Communications Commission all hold the belief that cell phones do not cause cancer, stating that there is no strong scientific evidence to show causality. Three major studies, the Interphone, the Danish study, and the Million Women Study, all found no increase in brain cancer with cell phone use. Only two smaller studies found an association. The CERENAT study out of France found that heavy users of cell phones did have an increased risk of both gliomas and meningiomas. Another study from Sweden saw statistically significant trends of increasing brain cancer risk for long durations and many years of cell phone use, especially among people who began using cell phones before age 20. So, again the studies have inconsistent findings and are not clear.

Regardless of whether or not cell phones actually cause cancer, we can all avoid some of the radiation from phones by using some precautionary measures.

* Keeping phones away from our heads is an important first step. When making a phone call, you can use a Bluetooth headset. You should be aware that wireless Bluetooth devices also give off radiation, but to a lesser degree. You can also use an ear piece or ear buds with a cord that is attached to the phone. This allows you to hear the caller directly into your ear and to speak into a microphone in close proximity to your mouth. These do not give off any radiation since they are corded.

* Texting is also another great option. I know I personally often prefer to text rather than to have a conversation on the phone simply for the time and convenience factor.

* If you do need to make a phone call, use the phone's built-in speaker. This allows you to hear the other person, and vice versa, without putting the phone up to your ear.

* Many newer model cars also have a built-in Bluetooth system. You can easily connect your phone to your to the car and receive or make phone calls through the stereo system.

* At night, if you can turn off your phone, it will do wonders. Not only will it stop the transmission of radio waves, but it will also give you a

probably much-needed break from technology and light emitted from your device. Many times we are tempted to look at our phones when we wake up, whether it be during the night or first thing in the morning. Breaking that habit can be great for our psyche.

* Do not wear your phone. This is probably more difficult for men than women. Women tend to carry cell phones in their purses or other bags. Men tend to carry them in a pocket. Although clothing will create a barrier, be cognizant to move the phone around if you must carry it on your body ... perhaps from a front pocket to a back pocket, from the jacket to a belt clip. And women should never carry it in their bra. The fatty tissue of the breast readily absorbs the radiation from the phone, potentially fostering tumor growth. When possible, put your cell phone on a table or in a brief case or bag when you do not need it on your person.

* Do your research when selecting a phone case as well. Look at the manufacturer's website or reviews of the cell phone case. Some are designed to limit your exposure to radiation. However, others that are designed to prevent damage to the phone (i.e., cracks, dents, etc.) may actually *increase* the amount of radiation. This happens because cases can weaken the signal by blocking the antenna and causing the phone to work harder to establish a connection. These types of cases tend to be thicker and denser.

* If you have young children, limit their use of cell phones. Children should not be making phone calls often, especially with phones near their little heads. Even excessive game playing on cell phones should be

avoided. Children's thinner skulls and bones allow them to absorb twice the amount of radiation as a grown-up. One study found that a cell phone call lasting only two minutes causes brain hyperactivity in children that persists for an hour.

11) Unnecessary CT Scans

Sometimes it becomes medically necessary to obtain scans. CT scans are a great diagnostic tool, but they deliver much more radiation than x-rays and may be overused, says Barton Kamen, MD, PhD, chief medical officer for the Leukemia & Lymphoma Society. In fact, researchers suggest that one-third of CT scans could be unnecessary. CT scans are a form of ionizing radiation, which if you'll remember, is a much riskier exposure than that of non-ionizing radiation. High doses of this radiation can trigger leukemia.

Researchers at the National Cancer Institute estimate that 29,000 future cancer cases could be attributed to the 72 million CT scans performed in the country each year. A 2009 study of medical centers in the San Francisco Bay Area also calculated an elevated risk: one extra case of cancer for every 400 to 2,000 routine chest CT exams.

People who have CT procedures as children may be at higher risk because children are more sensitive to radiation and have a longer life expectancy than adults. Women are also at a somewhat higher risk than men of developing cancer after receiving the same radiation exposures at the same ages.

That being said, *not* having the procedure can be much more risky than having it, especially if CT is being used to diagnose cancer or another serious condition in someone who has signs or symptoms of disease. You and your doctor must weigh your options and determine if the scan is necessary. Make sure scans are not repeated if you see multiple doctors, and ask if another test, such as an ultrasound or MRI, could substitute.

In 2010, the U.S. Food and Drug Administration (FDA) launched the "Initiative to Reduce Unnecessary Radiation Exposure from Medical Imaging." This initiative focuses on the safe use of medical imaging devices, informed decision-making about when to use specific imaging procedures, and increasing patients' awareness of their radiation exposure. In conjunction, the American College of Radiology (ACR) has developed the ACR Appropriateness Criteria, evidence-based guidelines to help providers make appropriate imaging and treatment decisions for a number of clinical conditions. So, safety measures are being taken, but you, as a patient and consumer, still need to ultimately be in charge of your healthcare.

12) Smoking

This is a no-brainer. Everyone knows that smoking and other tobacco-based products are harmful to one's health. That being said, millions of people are still smoking, largely because of the addictive nature of tobacco.

Tobacco contains nicotine which is a stimulant and highly addictive drug. It is very quickly absorbed into the bloodstream. It causes the brain to release adrenaline, creating a buzz of pleasure and energy. The buzz fades quickly though, leading to tiredness and irritability. This feeling is what makes a person light up the next cigarette. Since the body is able to build up a high tolerance to nicotine, more and more cigarettes are needed in order to get the nicotine's pleasurable effects and prevent withdrawal symptoms.

According to the World Health Organization, it's estimated that 1.1 billion people smoke worldwide. That is about one in every three adults. The world's largest producer and consumer of cigarettes is China.

In the United States, about 15% of the population smokes, which is about 36 million people. The CDC states that cigarette smoking is the leading cause of preventable disease and death in the United States, accounting for more than 480,000 deaths every year, or one of every five deaths.

A host of illnesses are associated with smoking as it can harm just about every organ in the body. Smoking causes about 90% of lung cancer cases. It also is known to cause COPD (Chronic Obstructive Pulmonary Disease) which inhibits proper oxygen exchange in the lungs and can also cause death. Smoking increases the risk of heart and cardiovascular disease. It's also associated with an increased risk of stroke.

Besides lung cancer, smoking also causes or contributes to a host of other cancers. The following is a short list of those cancers: bladder, cervical, leukemia, colorectal, esophageal, kidney, larynx, liver, oropharyngeal (mouth, throat, tonsils, and soft palate), pancreatic, stomach, and tracheal.

Chewing tobacco is also linked with cancer, especially that of the mouth, esophagus, and pancreas. Smoking cigars is also associated with cancer risk. Cigar smoking causes cancer of the oral cavity, larynx, esophagus, and lung. It may also cause cancer of the pancreas. Moreover, daily cigar smokers, particularly those who inhale, are at increased risk for developing heart disease and other types of lung disease.

If you smoke or chew tobacco, it is of utmost importance to try to quit. Once you stop smoking, cancer risk drops in half after five years. The American Lung Association has a host of resources to help with smoking cessation. Groups like "Freedom From Smoking" and "Quitter's Circle" provide support in person and online. Doctors can also prescribe medication to effectively help with quitting. It's not an easy addiction to break, but quitting will certainly add years to your life.

Final Thoughts on Environmental Toxins to Avoid

After reading this chapter, you now know that toxins are all around you. (We've touched on a few major ones, but there are a host of others.) Hopefully you also understand there is no earthly way to avoid them all. You might not even really *want* to do that. Personally, I will continue to occasionally get gel manicures. I'm certainly not giving up my cell phone. And who doesn't love some scented lotions and body washes? However, knowing the risks associated with environmental toxins allows me to make informed decisions. I can limit my use of them even if I don't give them up completely.

We can't live our lives worrying about exposure, but we can arm ourselves with information. Awareness is key. You, too, may be able to limit the frequency and duration with which you come into contact with toxins. You can buy organic cosmetics, toiletries, and cleaning supplies. You can limit your use of other hazardous materials like VOCs. You can refuse CT scans or only get them when absolutely necessary. You can stop smoking and lovingly encourage others you know to do the same.

It's all about taking control of our health. All of us are living with environmental toxins in our bodies and, for many of us, these toxins may be causing us to be ill and to seek medical care. Limiting the amount of internal pollutants allows our bodies and our livers to focus on doing their jobs unburdened. In the next chapter, we'll also look at some effective ways to detoxify our bodies, to get rid of some of those poisons. This is so helpful because the cause of most health problems is either due to a buildup of toxins or a deficiency of nutrients. We need to nourish our bodies inside and out. Remember, our bodies really are our temples. Without a healthy and sound structure, we can't enjoy life as it was meant to be.

* Anticancer Action *

Make this simple, non-toxic cleaner and use it to sanitize your kitchen and bathrooms:

1 cup water

1 cup vinegar

10-20 drops essential oil (lemon, eucalyptus, or tea tree work well)

Pour each into a glass spray bottle and shake to combine.

Chapter 7: Ways to Detoxify

Our bodies are inundated with toxins. They come from our environment in the form of fragrances, household beauty products, and cleaning supplies. They enter our mouths through processed, packaged food and from non-organic, pesticide-ridden and GMO food. Heck, toxins are even in our drinking water and the air we breathe. We cannot avoid them. We can do our best to limit our exposure through eating better or choosing to use more natural cleaning and beauty supplies. But our bodies still crave a break and need a way to release stored toxins so that they don't make us ill or lead to diseases like cancer.

It's important to note that our bodies have built-in detox mechanisms, and they're inherently always detoxifying to a certain extent. Our kidneys and colons help to eliminate waste through urine and feces respectively. Our lungs filter out toxins and debris from the air we breathe. Our skin is our largest organ, and it eliminates toxins through sweat. Our skin can also show us when we might have compromised detoxification if we see rashes, acne, or other sores. Our livers also act as primary filters for toxins. The lymph system collects unwanted "debris" in the body such as fats, bacteria, and other harmful materials and filters them through the lymph nodes. So, although our bodies can eliminate unwanted toxins, sometimes we require a bit of help to boost that process, especially if we're filled with and surrounded by environmental toxins. This is where detoxes come into play.

Our body can sometimes signal to us that it needs a little extra help with detoxification. The following are some signs that you may benefit from a detox:

* bloating
* increased belly fat and/or weight loss resistance
* sinus congestion
* sugar cravings
* white-coated tongue
* acne or rosacea
* rash or itchy skin
* chemical sensitivity (especially to smells)
* inability to handle small amounts of alcohol
* insomnia

Detoxifying can help eliminate the junk from our bodies and bloodstream. Its benefits include improving immunity, soothing achy muscles and joints, supporting weight loss, stabilizing blood sugars, boosting energy, decreasing pain and inflammation, reducing intestinal issues, clearing the mind, and cleaning up the skin. Detoxes also help reverse the aging process, and who doesn't want to feel and look younger? Best of all, this is something we can do simply and at home.

Detoxifying the body doesn't need to be a scary form of deprivation. We don't have to suffer, starve, or take expensive trips to health spas.

Many forms and variations of detoxes exist. Some are easier to follow than others. Some give greater results. However, any of them can be beneficial. Continue reading to discover just some of the possible ways to detox. You can choose one or two (or several) that are best for you, pique your interest, and seem attainable. Know that most major dietary detoxes are only to be used for a short amount of time, so we're not committing ourselves to lengthy lifestyle changes. Major detoxes can be used once or twice a year to achieve great results. Other mini-detox tricks can be used daily or weekly, so if you're not up for big changes, little changes can still yield good results.

1) Dry Brushing

Let's start with something very simple. Dry brushing is essentially brushing your skin typically using a medium-soft, natural-bristle brush. (We'll get to the technique in a moment.) The premise behind dry brushing is primarily to help rid the skin and bloodstream of toxins by encouraging cell turnover and circulation.

You can find these brushes at most general merchandise stores or bath supply stores. Having a brush with a longer handle is useful in getting to hard to reach places like your back.

The brushes are designed to gently exfoliate, improve circulation, condition skin, and boost the lymphatic system. It's also said to sweep away dead skin cells, improve digestion, improve the appearance of cellulite, and help the cells, and the body in general, remove waste. Dry brushing is preferred over wet brushing because you can remove surface skin cells easier and the brush tends to slide over skin easier when it's dry.

To dry brush, start at your feet and brush upward towards the heart. The chest area is where the lymph system drains. Always aim to brush toward the heart so that toxins are moved into circulation and eliminated through the lymph system. Next, move to your arms. Start at your fingers and brush upward. Use firm, small strokes upwards, or work in a circular motion. Brush your abdomen in a circular fashion as well. Using the long handle, reach over your shoulder and brush your back upwards from the bottom and downwards from the shoulders. Never put too much pressure. The effect is to gently exfoliate and/or promote circulation, not to scratch the skin. Your skin should only turn a little pink or reddish depending on your natural skin color. Do this for three to five minutes. Then, take a shower afterward. This helps to rinse away dead skin cells and further stimulate circulation.

Dry brushing is pretty darn relaxing and feels so good, especially when skin is dry and itchy. It's a quick way to treat yourself every day.

2) Massage

Everyone deserves a massage now and again. Yes, it can be costly depending on where you go, but it's worthwhile, even if you only get massages occasionally.

Why are massages so good for us? First, massages do the obvious: they help us relax and get rid of muscle stiffness. This is why most people seek massage therapy. But as an added bonus, like dry brushing, massages also help to eliminate toxins from our bodies. Trained massage therapists push on pressure points, and they also find places where you have lactic acid build up. These are the typical spots where toxins have built up and where you may experience some pain as a result. By rubbing these areas, toxins are released from stored body tissue. Drinking plenty of water after a massage helps to expel those toxins through urination.

If you can't afford a massage, have a partner or loved one give you a massage. This is a very cost effective way to reap the benefits. And if that person is a significant other, that feel-good hormone oxytocin can be released into your bloodstream. Win, win!

When I was a nurse in the hospital, one of my favorite acts of kindness was to give my patients a back rub. And boy, did that make their days too! Especially when someone is ill, massage can help promote lymphatic drainage and increase circulation, helping the person heal quicker.

If you add essential oils to massage oils or lotion, you'll be getting some added bonuses. Incorporating essential oils can encourage the body to further remove toxic waste. Some oils that are thought to help with the detoxification process include lavender, fennel, oregano, juniper, ginger, orange, lemon, lemongrass, peppermint, and grapefruit.

3) Epsom Salt Baths

Epsom salt baths can provide stress-relief and promote relaxation. This is due to their rich magnesium content. We'll look at this more in-depth in Chapter 9. However, Epsom salts also work to effectively detoxify the body. Human skin is a highly porous membrane. By adding minerals like magnesium and sulfate (Epsom salt) to your bathwater, it triggers a process called reverse osmosis. This actually pulls salt out of your body and harmful toxins along with it.

To draw a detoxifying bath, pour one to two cups of Epsom salts into your bath water. Aim to soak for 30-40 minutes. This ensures both that the toxins are pulled out of the body and that the minerals from the water are absorbed. Also, try to hydrate by drinking a large glass of water afterward. This will further help to eliminate toxins and make sure you're not becoming dehydrated from the salt pulling.

Those who are already ill with cancer can benefit too. Taking Epsom salt baths daily can help relieve symptoms of the illness and also reduce anxiety and irritability and improve sleep patterns. Other benefits of these baths are relief of constipation (thank magnesium for that); absorption of sulfates for joint, skin, and nerve tissue health; reduction of inflammation; and liver detox (thanks to the sulfur in sulfates) which rids the body of toxins from foods, medications, etc. You could also add some essential oils to your bath (see "massage" section above). These increase the detoxifying effects and further promote relaxation.

4) Neti Pots

Neti pots became popular a few years back, especially after they were featured on Dr. Oz. However, they've been around for centuries and used in Ayurvedic medicine. A Neti pot looks like a small tea pot with a long spout, like an Aladdin's lamp. It is used for nasal irrigation. A saline solution or salt-based powder is mixed with warm water. A person uses the pot by placing the end of the spout in one nostril, tilting the head toward the other side so the nostril in use is up, and leans over a sink. The warm liquid enters through the upper nostril, irrigates the sinuses, and comes out through the other nostril.

Nasal irrigation can alleviate symptoms of colds, sinus problems, and nasal allergies. It rinses away dust, pollen, and environmental irritants. It supports a healthy upper respiratory tract. It improves the condition of the cilia (little hair-like structures inside the nose) and their ability to remove bacteria. By using a Neti pot, you can prevent infections from entering your body through the nasal passages and/or stop infections from getting worse. By removing toxins, the nasal passage is cleared and the immune system can rest. Viruses and bacteria can be washed away before they colonize and infect the body.

To prevent infection from the pot itself, always use distilled, sterile, or previously boiled water. Tap water can harbor bacteria. It's also important to add salt to the water. Most Neti pots come with pre-made powder packets that you'll mix into the warm water. This saline solution has the same salt-to-water balance as your natural bodily tissues, making it safer and more comfortable for irrigation. Also, it's important to properly care for your Neti pot. Either wash the device thoroughly by hand, or put it in the dishwasher if it's dishwasher-safe. Make sure you dry it thoroughly as well to prevent bacteria form harboring in wet areas.

5) Acupuncture

Acupuncture is a holistic health technique that stems from Traditional Chinese Medicine practices. It involves having a trained specialist insert tiny needles into your body at the source of pain or into "blocked" zones. You might be thinking, "Ouch!" Surprisingly, because the needles are so thin, acupuncture is relatively pain-free.

Acupuncture helps to unclog these blocked zones and to release the toxins naturally. It is said to flush out toxins by stimulating Qi flow through the vital detoxification organs. If the organs of elimination are open, acupuncture may push the liver to detoxify more. It's also thought to activate the spleen for better immune response and to facilitate bowel movements to help with elimination of toxins.

Acupuncture has been known to help people detox from drug addiction, too. Patients claim that acupuncture reduces cravings, eases withdrawal and physical pain, and decreases anxiety. For the general population, acupuncture may help to detox organs, encourage better sleep, improve chronic pain, reduce headaches and migraines, and even prevent cognitive decline.

6) Chiropractic Care

Chiropractic care is often used in conjunction with massage. It works to detoxify the body in similar ways. It is a natural form of health care that uses spinal adjustments to correct misalignments and restore proper function to the nervous system, helping the body to heal naturally. When someone visits a chiropractor (who is also trained in nutrition, by the way), they are having their spine and accompanying bones or joints "manipulated." After the spine's vertebrae are put back into proper alignment, the nervous system (stemming from the spinal cord) is better able to perform its job. Since the central nervous system can then work correctly, it sends the message to the rest of the body to rid itself of toxins. In fact, sometimes after an adjustment, people may feel a bit woozy or sick. This is actually thought to be related to the release of toxins, and the feeling usually passes fairly quickly. Like with massage, drinking lots of fluids afterward can help.

From personal experience, I can tell you that chiropractic care is wonderful for treating recurrent headaches and neck pain related to scoliosis. After the adjustment, my chiropractor also applies TENS (transcutaneous electrical nerve stimulation) units to areas of pain. These are small electrodes that are applied to the skin via adhesive pads. Currents travel through electrodes and into the skin stimulating specific nerve pathways to produce a tingling or massaging sensation that reduces the perception of pain. Let me tell you, this is relaxation at its best! After about 15-20 minutes of TENS treatment, I lie on a roller bed. This is essentially a massage from underneath. The rollers move from your head to your toes and back again, over and over. I leave these appointments feeling like a new woman. I've never experienced sickness afterward, but often I do feel quite relaxed and sleepy.

Besides realignment, chiropractic care is reported to help improve ear infections; back, head, neck, and joint pain; scoliosis; sciatica; constipation; asthma; blood pressure; organ function; and arthritis. It may also lessen the deteriorating side effects of diseases like MS.

Research has shown that it also reduces inflammatory cytokines, boosts the immune system, decreases oxidative stress, and improves energy. A study published in the *Journal of Manipulative and Physiological Therapeutics* found that spinal manipulation decreased inflammatory cytokines, especially in the two hours following the adjustment. This suggests that regular chiropractic adjustments would be beneficial in reducing overall inflammation.

7) Yoga

Yoga helps to detox not only your body but your mind as well. As you move through the various yoga poses, you build strength and flexibility. By stretching your joints and muscles, you can release stored toxins. You'll also sweat, especially if you're engaging in hot yoga. We'll get into benefits of sweat for detoxification later.

Yoga also incorporates pranayama breathing. This is a yogic breathing exercise that has the ability to quickly increase energy, release stress, improve mental clarity, and improve physical health. It is the formal practice of controlling the breath, which is the source of our prana, or vital life force. This deep breathing releases stress, calms the body and mind, reduces blood pressure, and relaxes muscles as well. Deep breathing exercises help clear out toxins that may have built up in the lungs which can help improve lung performance and clear airways. It gets more nourishing oxygen into the body. Blood that is rich in oxygen helps you feel better and gives you more energy. Deep breathing also reaches the deepest depths of your lungs and helps to expel and break up residue.

Yoga improves circulation and cardiovascular output. This, in turn, stimulates the lymph system, helping to move toxins into circulation and out of the body.

Some believe that certain yoga positions that involve twisting or inversion can literally wring out toxins from your organs. There's no scientific literature to prove this, but it's an interesting idea. If nothing else, yoga increases your flexibility. A 2009 study in the *American Journal of Physiology* showed that for people age 40 and over, flexibility in the body was accompanied by flexibility in the arteries, reducing the risk for cardiovascular disease and even death.

Yoga can also encourage good nutrition, as one feels longer and leaner afterward. Studies have also shown that yoga has a beneficial impact on leptin, helping the body control appetite.

A 2013 study in Norway found that regular practice of gentle yoga and meditation had a rapid effect at the genetic level in circulating cancer-fighting immune cells. So it appears yoga really does strengthen the body and mind.

8) Other Exercise

There is nothing better than a good sweat. It makes you feel you've worked hard, and it literally cleanses you from the inside out. When you exercise, you may just be sweating out toxins. When you hydrate after a good workout, you are also helping to flush out additional toxins through the kidneys.

Deep breathing associated with cardiovascular exercise also helps the lungs to eliminate toxins. Strong exhalations can empty the lungs of unneeded carbon dioxide and allow for a deeper fresh breath of more oxygenated air.

Exercise encourages circulation, too. In general, circulation equals better health because the entire body is being flooded with oxygen-rich blood. Moving the body helps to circulate both blood and lymph. The more they circulate, the more the liver and lymph nodes can do the job of cleansing and purifying the blood and lymph.

Exercise can also encourage weight loss. Toxic substances are stored in body fat. So, it follows that a decrease in body fat can also eliminate unwanted toxins.

So what kind of exercise is best for detoxification? Anything that gets the heart pumping, the lungs breathing deeply, and allows you to sweat a bit. That can be simply taking a brisk walk or engaging in some circuit training or weight lifting.

9) Saunas

Saunas have been used by societies for thousands of years. The word sauna is an ancient Finnish word meaning bathhouse. In Finland, there are millions of saunas, at least two million according to official registers. In fact, most homes and summer houses have a sauna, often built-in but also sometimes detached from the main home as an actual bath house. Saunas are a warm and welcome past-time in the very cold climate of Finland. Being 50% Finnish, this is personally fascinating to me. I remember hearing stories about these bathhouses from my grandfather and other relatives. My father, a Lutheran pastor, served at a Finnish-Lutheran church (in the United States), and in the parsonage was a built-in sauna. Finns love their saunas!

Finns say the sauna is a poor man's pharmacy, curing many ailments. Using saunas, for detoxification or for therapeutic reasons, involves sitting in a small room designed as a place to experience dry or wet heat sessions. (Typically, you think of saunas as dry heat and steam rooms as wet heat.) Temperatures can reach 212 °F (or 100 °C). In the United States, Underwriters Laboratory (UL) dictates that the maximum temperature at ceiling level is 194° F (90° C). Although this seems exceedingly high, by controlling the humidity (10% or lower), the dry heat allows people to sit in a sauna for periods of time. Temperature and humidity are controlled by the user by pouring water onto hot stones.

There are two main types of saunas: conventional and infrared. The conventional was described above. Infrared saunas are typically set at a lower temperature, between 120 and 140° F. Infrared rays heat the body directly and the air secondarily. There is no humidity at all in these saunas.

Whether using conventional or infrared sauna, the goal is perspiration, and a lot of it. Sweating has been proven to effectively flush toxins out of the system while maintaining optimum health of the body. According to Net Physician, the benefits of sauna therapy include detoxification of the body, anti-viral activity, weight loss, pain relief, sinus relief, improved circulation, relaxation, and skin conditioning. Therapeutic sauna has been shown to aid adaptation, reduce stress hormones, lower blood pressure, and improve cardiovascular conditions.

Although saunas are healthy for most, there are contraindications for some people. Anyone with acute heart disease is typically advised to avoid saunas, especially anyone with a recent heart attack. Those with very low or very high blood pressure might also want to consult their doctor before using a sauna. The heat taxes the heart and circulatory system a bit, increasing heart rate by up to 30 beats per minute. Alcohol consumption during sauna bathing increases the risk of hypotension, arrhythmia, and sudden death, and should be avoided. Some medications like diuretics, beta-blockers, or barbiturates may also cause an ill-effect, so asking a doctor in advance is a good idea. The very young and the elderly should limit sauna use to only a few minutes at a time, and definitely no more than 15 minutes. Pregnant women should typically also avoid saunas.

10) Colon Cleanses

Our colons eliminate stool that's made up of a combination of bacteria, water, unused nutrients, unneeded electrolytes, and digested or undigested food. The stool also carries toxins out of our bodies. Regular bowel movements are immensely important for colon health and for normal detoxification. If someone is not having daily bowel movements, colon cleanses may be an important strategy to incorporate.

Different types of colon cleanses exist. One type requires that a professional perform the cleanse (colonic), while others involve using a solution (enema) or supplement (laxative) at home. Many colon cleanses work by inserting a tube into the rectum followed by large amounts of water, which makes its way through the colon. The water carries out any matter that might be dry and lodged in place. When done safely, colon cleanses are safe and effective. These should be done no more than once a week.

Other ways to cleanse the colon involve eating high fiber foods, fermented foods, and taking probiotics and probiotics. If these do not work to increase frequency of bowel movements, other methods of colon cleansing may be beneficial.

Dietary Detoxes

Dietary detoxes typically involve removing certain foods or food groups from one's daily diet. Sometimes they can also involve incorporating more of a certain food in lieu of other, less desirable foods or beverages. A good detox insists on highly nourishing, vitamin-rich substances and shuns chemical-laden, nutrient-poor, processed junk. Some detoxes can be short. For example, some may last for two or three days. Others may be lifestyle alterations that can be used for a lifetime. The goal is to give our bodies a break from foods and drinks that can be toxic or burden our systems.

In this section, we'll look at some sustainable or, at least, attainable ways to detox. There are hundreds of fad diets and detoxes on the market and/or with popular online followings, but many of those may be unsafe or have unpleasant side effects. Continue reading to learn about a few "healthier" dietary detox strategies geared to do more good than harm.

1) Increasing Clean Water Consumption

Water is nature's way of flushing toxins out of the body. Water allows your kidneys to filter toxins, helps your cells take in nutrients and remove waste, and transports nutrients to every organ in your body. If you don't drink enough water, then you might be suffering from a buildup of toxins throughout your body and may be compromising your immune system.

In a study conducted at the Centre for Human Nutrition at the University of Sheffield, England, researchers concluded that women who stay adequately hydrated reduce their risk of breast cancer by 79%. Another study, done at the Fred Hutchinson Cancer Research Center in Seattle, found that women who drink more than five glasses of water a day have a 45% reduced risk of colon cancer compared with women who drink two or fewer glasses of water a day.

Unfortunately, most of us really don't drink enough pure, filtered water. We drink coffee, juices, sodas, but not enough water. In Chapter 3, we discussed how even tap water consumption should be limited or avoided due to harmful chemicals. So, how much good quality, filtered water do we actually need?

We've all heard drinking eight glasses of water per day is a great starting point. This allows the kidneys and other waste organs to function normally. However, you may need significantly more when it comes to detoxifying the body. A good rule of thumb is to drink about 90 ounces of water throughout the day if you are focusing on detoxification specifically. This amounts to at least five or six standard-sized bottles (500 ml or 16.9 oz) of filtered water per day. Others recommend drinking half of your weight in ounces. For example, a 200 pound person would aim to drink about 100 ounces; a 150 pound person would aim for 75 ounces. Thus, the amount will vary based on gender, body size, and weight. Consumption of water should be spaced out throughout the day.

It is possible to go overboard, however. Too much water can throw off your electrolyte balance and cause things like hyponatremia (low salt levels) which in turn causes nausea, confusion, headaches, and fatigue.

Often, athletes or even kids who play sports may turn to drinks like Gatorade or other electrolyte-rich beverages to replace salt. These, however, may not be the best option. They are typically filled with sugar and/or sugar substitutes. In Chapter 2, we talked about the benefits of drinking lemon water with Himalayan sea salt. Adding a pinch of sea salt to lemon water is a great option for hydrating without losing any electrolytes. If you'll remember, Himalayan sea salt is rich in trace minerals, so you'll be getting hydration as well as nourishment. Try doing this a few times a day, perhaps once first thing in the morning and then later in the afternoon or after any strenuous exercise.

Drinking hot lemon water (with or without sea salt) first thing in the morning is a great way to detoxify the body. When you drink it on an empty stomach, it can help to detox the body before any other process like digestion begins. It helps flush the digestive system and rehydrate the body. The lemon provides vitamin C, assists the liver in producing enzymes and releasing toxins, is antibacterial, helps elicit bowel movements, and stimulates stomach acid and bile production. The warmth of the water also aids in digestion, assists with flushing out toxins, and increases blood flow which helps with detoxification.

2) Juice/Smoothie Cleanses

Juicing has become a popular trend. Juice and smoothie stores are popping up everywhere. At-home juicers are a market fad, some quite expensive and others more affordable. Whether you make your own or buy them, drinking juices can be a therapeutic form of detox.

Essentially, juicing extracts the juice from fresh fruits or vegetables. The resulting liquid contains most of the vitamins, minerals and plant chemicals (phytonutrients) found in the whole fruit. The pulp and fiber have been removed.

Juicing is a great way to get lots of vegetables and fruits into your diet. It's also a way to incorporate produce you might never have tried. Most of us purchase the same few fruits and veggies we're used to eating to prepare at home. But juicing gives you the freedom to try new varieties without having to hunt down recipes.

Juice cleanses are controversial, however. If you're only consuming juice, you're missing out on the fiber that accompanies fruits and vegetables in their natural states. Juices can end up elevating blood sugar since they have none of the fiber to balance the sudden intake of fructose.

There are a lot of pros to juicing, too. It can give the digestive system a break. It assists in resting and repairing the gut. Consuming phytonutrient-dense, plant-based juices allows food to be assimilated quickly through the intestines. This consumes less energy, and allows the nutrient-dense food to repair the gut. It cleanses the liver, giving it a break from toxins in other foods. Juices also eliminate most known food allergy and sensitivity triggers like gluten, dairy, and soy. Using organic fruits and veggies allows the body's mitochondria to create energy without having to fight off a plethora of free radicals and inflammation.

Juice cleanses can be done as a "fast" or just incorporated into your existing diet. There are some warnings you should consider if you're thinking of doing a juice-only fast. Typically a one to three day fast, for most people, is just fine. However, if you're experiencing lightheadedness, nausea, headaches, low blood sugars, or mood swings, you should quit the fast. Juice-only fasts are low in protein and calories which could contribute to feelings of fatigue. Juice fasts are not recommended for people with diabetes and for pregnant or nursing mothers.

I think the addition of juices to your daily regimen could be quite beneficial. If you're inclined, I believe a one to two day reset with a juice fast could also help. I personally prefer drinking **smoothies** because the fiber remains along with the vitamins and minerals. (These are typically made with a blender or similar device rather than a juicer which eliminates the pulp and fiber.) This is helpful in stimulating waste elimination through the colon. In fact, I begin every day with a smoothie. Mine are rich in veggies and fruit (like bananas, frozen pineapple or berries, frozen broccoli, and spinach), but I also typically include some protein powder as well. This is my daily breakfast, and it keeps me full for hours.

Probably the most important thing to consider when juicing is that your produce is organic. You do not want to add in toxic pesticides when you're attempting to detox. It defeats the purpose because your body must then work to mitigate the toxic burden, stressing it further. Remember the "dirty dozen" we looked at in Chapter 2? Consuming those 12 fruits and vegetables in their organic form is always best.

3) Sugar Detoxes

One effective way to reduce burdens on the body is to try a sugar detox. There are programs on the market if you're looking for guidance. A favorite is *The 21-Day Sugar Detox* book by Diane Sanfilippo. The author leads you through a whole-foods nutrition plan to reset your body and reduce sugar cravings. The benefit of programs like this is that there are online support groups to help guide you and answer questions. However, you can effectively do a sugar detox alone.

So what is a sugar detox? Basically, for a period of time, you avoid any foods (and condiments) that come in a box, package, or can or that have a label. This is because processed foods typically contain sugars or sweeteners or break down as sugars in the body. All refined sugars are avoided in food or beverages as well. This means no candy, cookies, sweet treats, sodas, etc. Most grains, especially white rice and white flours are also avoided. Some stricter versions also warn against consuming high-sugar fruits like bananas or pineapple, but berries and green apples may be eaten. Fruit juices and dried fruit are also "no-nos". Alcohol should be eliminated during a detox as well. Some detoxes recommend consuming no dairy either, as milk and milk products inherently contain sugars and are also sources of inflammation for most people.

Instead, you stick to real, whole, fresh food. Vegetables, low-sugar fruits, meats and fish, eggs, nuts and seeds (without oils and sugars), and even some dark chocolate are all permitted.

Why perform a sugar detox? Our bodies are burdened by sugar. Sugar makes us fat and sick. Incidentally, most sugar consumed in the US is not organic and is derived from GMO, pesticide-ridden sugarcane. Sugar stresses the liver. The liver must process all of the excess sugar we eat, and since we typically eat it in abundance, the liver can't use it all for energy and instead turns it into fat. Have you heard of Non-Alcoholic Fatty Liver Disease? It's a real phenomenon and related directly to sugar and simple carbohydrate consumption. Remember, we need our liver for normal detoxification and blood filtration, so if it is burdened by processing excess sugar, it cannot appropriately do its job. We also know of sugar's relationship with Type 2 Diabetes, obesity, cancer, and other illnesses.

An occasional break from sugar and processed foods may just be what your body craves. It's up to you how long to pursue the detox. Sugar detox programs typically last 20-30 days. However, even taking a break from these foods one to two days a week will help your body function more optimally. If you do decide to do longer detoxes (such as a month-long program), you may begin to break your sugar addiction for good. Your body will crave sweets less and less, and eating lower-sugar foods may become your new norm.

4) Elimination Diets

An elimination diet is not technically a detox, but it does help a person determine which foods trigger sensitivity and inflammation for them. We all know people who have food allergies. Perhaps someone's throat gets itchy or closes when they consume shellfish. Another person may develop hives or rashes when they eat eggs. These are more overt allergies that can be picked up a traditional blood test. This blood work tests for the presence of IgE antibodies. A skin prick test can do the same. These antibodies specifically elicit food allergy symptoms.

Some people, however, may have food sensitivities that are not picked up by this type of test. The difference between a food allergy and a food sensitivity is that, with a sensitivity, the person may not have an immediate reaction. A food sensitivity can cause inflammation in the body. In fact, many people have some form of sensitivity unbeknownst to them. Sensitivities can cause things like headaches, joint pain, fatigue, bloating, brain fog, runny nose, and insomnia. They are not life-threatening, but they are very common.

Let me give you an example. I've struggled with knee pain for years, since I was a little girl. I was a runner in high school and jogged for exercise well into my 30s. I chalked the knee pain up to the fact that running broke down my joints. To an extent this was true. However, for various reasons, I decided to have food sensitivity testing done and found that I was "highly reactive" to white potatoes. Wouldn't you know that when I eliminated them from my diet, my knee pain just about disappeared?

Food sensitivity testing is available, but may or may not be covered by insurance. This testing typically looks for IgG antibodies and different inflammatory markers. When I was tested for sensitivities I went through a naturopathic physician. The lab tests were out of pocket for me and ran about $300. Sure, that's not a drop in the bucket, but if you have any illnesses or ailments or are just curious about which foods might be causing underlying inflammation, it might be a good investment. One of the tests I had completed was called the MRT (Mediator Release Test). This is a patented test which looks for pro-inflammatory and proalgesic mediator releases from white cells. This involves cytokines, histamine, leukotrienes, prostaglandins, etc., from neutrophils, monocytes, eosinophils, and lymphocytes. The results of this test give you categories of reaction. For example, some foods are highly reactive, some moderately reactive, and some non-reactive. Each individual would yield different results. There are a myriad of other food sensitivity tests available. You can work with your medical doctor, functional medicine doctor (naturopath), or even a nutritionist to determine which testing might benefit you.

Even though testing can yield some helpful results, giving you a basis of information, they are not always 100% accurate. In my opinion, the best and most cost-effective way to determine if you have food sensitivities is to try an elimination diet. By removing possible irritants, the body may become less inflamed and begin to heal. When this happens, symptoms of inflammation like headaches, pains, rashes, gut disturbances, and even autoimmune conditions may go away. Essentially, this is a way to detox the body from foods that are specifically harmful to it. Again, just as each person's body chemistry is different, each person's trigger foods will be too. However, the most commonly irritating foods that should be avoided when doing an elimination diet are **gluten, soy, corn, peanuts, dairy, sugar, artificial sweeteners, eggs, and alcohol**. This will include most packaged and processed foods by definition.

An elimination diet should last for at least two weeks. However, according to some, elimination diets should be longer (about three to six weeks). It's believed that antibodies (the proteins your immune system makes when it negatively reacts to foods) take around three weeks to dissipate. So this is usually the minimum time needed for someone to fully heal from sensitives and to notice improvements in their symptoms.

5) Caffeine Detox

Caffeine is the number one drug of choice in the world. Millions of people, including myself (ahem), begin their day with the ritualistic practice of making a cup of Joe. We may add milk, creamer, sugar, coconut oil, MCT oil, or even butter. We've become coffee gourmands, making our creations that much more special and personalized. Coffee smells incredible, and it awakens your mind and senses. However, far too many of us are addicted to caffeine. We can't live without it. We can't even move in the morning until we've consumed our first cup. Sadly, caffeine is not a benign substance, and if consumed in excess, can harm our bodies.

Every once in a while, it's a good idea to get off the caffeine ... just to give our bodies a break and to see how we feel. Caffeine may be affecting us in negative ways that we might not associate it with. For one, caffeine stresses our adrenals glands, and adrenal fatigue can lead to overwhelming exhaustion. Caffeine also increases your stress hormones cortisol and epinephrine making you feel more stressed out, irritable, and anxious. Sometimes, we also use caffeine as a crutch when we don't get enough sleep. We think that because coffee helps us function, we are just fine sleeping less. We already know that sleep is absolutely crucial to our health and prevention of disease, so we cannot afford to skimp on it. Caffeine affects our neurotransmitters, interfering with serotonin and GABA, thus making us less happy and less calm. Those who suffer from stomach ailments or GERD (reflux), could also see an increase in symptoms because of caffeine. Some other "hidden" ailments attributed to caffeine are cystic breasts, increased blood pressure, osteoporosis, and headaches.

In Chapter 2, we discussed the benefits of coffee, so we don't need to avoid it completely. However, just an occasional break could be helpful if someone is symptomatic (fatigue, irritability, low moods, little sleep, heartburn, etc.) to see whether or not avoiding the substance could be beneficial.

Coffee is not the only beverage that contains caffeine. Some teas contain caffeine as well. Black, white, and green teas have varying levels of caffeine. According to the Mayo Clinic, brewed coffee contains 75-200 mg of caffeine; black tea has 14-70 mg; and green tea has 24-45 mg. White tea contains about 30-55 mg. The amount of caffeine content in tea depends upon the manufacturer's makeup of the tea, time brewed, and size of beverage. Of course there are other caffeinated beverages on the market.

Sodas can contain up to 100 mg of caffeine, and energy drinks can top out at over 300 mg! Also, be aware that even chocolate contains caffeine, so you'll need to watch out for those sweet treats, too.

Giving up caffeine, even if only for a brief period of time, can result in unpleasant side effects. One might experience caffeine withdrawal headaches. Other symptoms can be fatigue, irritability, lethargy, poor focus and concentration, insomnia, and even flu-like symptoms. It's best to gradually decrease the amount of caffeine in your diet. For example, if you normally drink two cups of coffee each morning, try to first drink one or one and a half cups for a few days. A few days later, reduce that to only one cup or a half cup, etc. You'll work your way down to eliminating caffeine completely. A slow withdrawal will help lessen unwanted side effects.

What should you drink instead? If you typically begin your day with coffee, try replacing it with warm lemon water. In Chapter 2, we discussed the benefits of lemon water sprinkled with Himalayan sea salt. This combination will revitalize you and give you lasting energy. You'll experience none of those crashes associated with caffeine withdrawal. Drink this combo during your 3:00 PM afternoon slump as well. Besides the natural change in circadian rhythms, often we become tired during this time due to dehydration and/or hypoglycemia. Lemon water with sea salt can help correct both problems. And best of all, it works as a flush for our system, aiding in detoxification.

Herbal teas are also a wonderful addition. Did you know you can actually get a lot of nourishment from herbal teas? They contain a host of antioxidants which further support detoxification pathways. Herbal teas are caffeine-free, but be sure to read labels in case the manufacturer combined the herbs with green or black tea, for example. Below are a few herbal teas that may help provide energy:

Ginger: Ginger stimulates circulation and the brain. It is also helpful for calming a queasy stomach.

Ginseng: Ginseng boosts your resilience to stress and helps with fatigue. It also helps with immunity.

Licorice: This is a delicious tea. If you don't like black licorice, don't worry. It doesn't contain the anise flavor. Licorice tea is actually quite sweet. It's helpful for anyone battling fatigue, especially adrenal fatigue from high stress. It stabilizes blood sugar, too.

Gingko Biloba: This tea increases blood-flow to the brain which improves concentration and memory-retention. It also helps fight off anxiety and depression.

Peppermint: Peppermint is often used to increase focus. It has a calming effect on the body as well, and it's soothing to the digestive tract.

Dandelion: Dandelion is somewhat bitter, but actually quite pleasant tasting. The taste is reminiscent of coffee, for those missing out on the taste. It is great for detoxification because it supports the liver and helps to remove toxins from the body.

Rosehip: Rosehip is known for rejuvenation of the mind and also the skin, as it contains vitamin C which has anti-aging properties. It has a refreshing, sweet taste.

Of course, each kind of herbal tea has its own benefits. There are hundreds from which to choose. You might experiment to find one or a combination that you enjoy.

The main caveat with drinking tea during a caffeine detox is that you do NOT want to do a "tea-tox." Tea-toxes are en vogue. You'll read of celebrities touting amazing weight loss claims. Tea-toxes often involve consuming teas that contain a laxative called senna. These can be addictive, but they can also harm your digestive tract and create serious side effects like cramping, diarrhea, nausea, fatigue, and dizziness. They are really not a safe form of detoxification, nor are they good for sustained weight loss. Long-term use can also alter the balance of electrolytes which can cause heart function disorders, muscle weakness, liver damage, and other harmful effects. So, stick with herbal teas.

5) Intermittent Fasting

Intermittent fasting (IF) gives the body a break from digesting food, allowing it to focus on detoxification. The liver can work on eliminating chemicals and toxins rather than aiding in digestion for period of time. When someone incorporates intermittent fasting, they eat the day's calories in a shorter time window. For example, a person may stop eating around 8:00 PM and not eat again until noon the next day. The remainder of the time, the person is fasting — only consuming water, black coffee, or unsweetened teas. This amounts to an eight-hour eating window. To be clear, a person would consume the same amount of calories per usual; they are just ingested during the eating window.

Intermittent fasting has many benefits beyond detoxification. It can help with insulin resistance. It allows the body to use fat as its primary source of energy instead of sugar since calories and carbohydrates are not entering the body. IF also improves the immune system by reducing free radical damage, regulating inflammatory conditions in the body, and even starving cancer cell formation. During a fast, the body can work at the cellular level to repair itself. IF has also been associated with longer lifespans, probably because of the aforementioned mechanisms. Earlier in the book, we mentioned Human Growth Hormone and that it is best when increased naturally. Well, IF promotes the increase of HGH, especially when someone exercises while in a temporarily fasted state.

Unlike prolonged fasting, IF can be incorporated into one's daily eating regimen. Many people use IF as a part of sustained weight loss. There are some contraindications to IF, however. Pregnant or nursing women should avoid it. Anyone with adrenal fatigue, cortisol disregulation, or low blood sugars should also consider eating more often. This is because IF is a stressor on the body, and those with cortisol imbalances can experience blood sugar swings and increased lethargy or brain fog. Anyone with a history of eating disorders should also be warned as fasting can trigger a return of disordered eating patterns and/or bingeing. There is some disagreement over whether diabetics should fast. Some say those with Type 2 diabetes may benefit from IF because the body uses fat instead of sugars for energy when fasting, and insulin sensitivity is improved. However, others warn of low blood sugar, especially for those taking exogenous insulin. So, if you are diabetic, consult your doctor before trying IF.

Prolonged fasting, fasting for longer periods of time, MUST be done very carefully. Some people might try fasting for one to three days. Others may go weeks without food. However, this is only something to try if you are in good health and really should be done in consultation with a doctor or naturopath. It is NOT something to incorporate regularly. Some people include longer fasts once or twice a year, but doing so more frequently is not advised as it does take a toll on the body. Prolonged fasting may be a good form of detoxification for some, but for many, it is not necessary and can actually be detrimental. For that reason, I believe intermittent fasting is the best choice for those wishing to experiment with fasting and/or for those who are looking for ways to lose weight and detoxify.

6) Ketogenic Diets

Simply stated, a ketogenic diet is an extremely low carb, moderate protein, and high fat diet. When a person begins to burn fat for fuel instead of carbohydrates and sugar, they enter into a state called "ketosis." Ketones are molecules produced in the liver from fat and used as alternative fuel when blood glucose is in short supply. Ketosis can also be accomplished when a person is fasting.

In a ketogenic diet, a person consumes no more than 10% of calories from carbohydrate and these are mostly in the form of green vegetables. Protein can range from 15-25% of caloric intake, and the remainder (70% or more) would be from fats. So, basically, a person focuses on eating healthy fats like coconut oil, olive oil, avocado, and butter. Nuts and seeds are acceptable in small amounts. Protein comes in the form of fatty fish, meat, eggs, and possibly some full-fat dairy. Carbohydrates are vegetable-based. Refined and processed carbs and grains are eliminated as are almost all fruits (some low-sugar fruits like berries, lemon, and green apples may be permitted). An example of a day's meal plan might be:

Breakfast: an omelet with spinach and bacon

Lunch: a chicken salad with olive oil and feta cheese

Dinner: a bunless, grass-fed beef burger topped with avocado and served with steamed, butter-coated vegetables

Ketogenic diets are not a "detox" per se, but they do give the body a break from processing sugar and help to eliminate the toxic burden refined foods place on the body. Being in ketosis has other health benefits, too.

Weight loss can occur effortlessly and rapidly. The body easily burns stored body fat instead of sugars. Those with Type 2 Diabetes can also benefit. Studies show that low-carbohydrate diets, which limit intake of sugar and processed grains, encourage improvements in the dyslipidemia of diabetes. Those taking insulin, however, need to consult a physician before attempting a ketogenic diet.

Ketogenic diets have been used to treat and even help reverse symptoms of cognitive impairments, including Alzheimer's symptoms. The brain can use fat for fuel, which is preferable in Alzheimer's disease, a disease also colloquially known as "Type 3 Diabetes." Essentially, sugars harm the brain.

Following a ketogenic diet may also help prevent and even kill cancer cells. A 2011 study published in the journal *Nutrition & Metabolism* found that mice in a ketotic state exhibited anti-tumor benefits. Researchers also stated, "Evidence exists that chronically elevated blood glucose, insulin and IGF1 levels facilitate tumorigenesis [creation of cancerous tumors] and worsen the outcome in cancer patients." So ketosis may be a way of warding off cancer by decreasing blood sugars and may also be an adjuvant to treatments like chemotherapy or radiation in patients with existing cancer.

If eating such a low-carb diet doesn't appeal to you, you can try carb cycling. This is when you alternate between higher carb and lower carb days. For the most benefit, experts recommend two high carb days a week with the remainder being low carb. However, even an "every other day" approach can be beneficial. On the higher carb days, you can consume some grains and fruit, but sugars and refined foods are still discouraged.

Higher carb days might include 150-300 grams of carbs. On the lower carb days, your body will reset and once again burn fat for fuel.

Because our bodies store toxins in fat cells, burning fat instead of sugar can release those toxins from stored body fat. They will then be taken to the liver to be processed and detoxed.

Final Thoughts on Ways to Detoxify

Our bodies perform detoxification every single day ... whether we consciously assist them or not. Our bodies crave the cleansing process as it allows for optimal functioning and health. However, with the amount of exposure to toxic chemicals, pesticides, and stress we face each day, sometimes our bodies become overwhelmed and can't keep up. Sometimes we need additional help to restore balance and expel unwanted waste.

Researchers have linked many sicknesses in industrialized countries to toxic build up in the body. Often, toxins bind to sex hormones or thyroid hormones which slows metabolism, causing weight gain. Additionally, toxins are stored in fat, making them systemic and long-lasting poisons. They begin to alter the very chemistry of our bodies and do damage at the cellular level. This can lead to disease and cancer. Detoxification is so important because it can literally reverse the symptoms of illness and change our lives.

In this chapter, we've perused some interesting detox strategies like dry brushing or Epsom salt baths that you can incorporate daily. You can start changing your life tomorrow just by drinking more filtered water, herbal teas, and green juices or smoothies. Simple changes and additions to your diet and lifestyle make a world of difference in improving your health.

If you're not ready for major dietary overhauls like ketogenic diets or intermittent or prolonged fasting, you can start by eating more organic foods. This removes the toxic burden of pesticides, hormones, and GMOs from the body. Eating a whole foods-based diet is another step. When we eat primarily from boxes and bags, we miss out on a great number of nutrients. But when we eat from nature, consuming fruits, vegetables, nuts and seeds, meat, and good oils like olive oil and coconut oil, we get that nourishment. And as an added bonus, our appetites are satiated because our bodies are getting what they need and desire. Cravings also go away. Eating processed foods literally starves our bodies, making us want to eat more in search of those necessary nutrients. Sugar robs our bodies of minerals and energy, too. It is our food supply's devil, causing illness, obesity, and literally killing us. So, at the very least, we should all reduce sugar in our daily diets.

Find a detoxification strategy that works for you. Try it for a few weeks (depending on what you've chosen) and see if you notice any improvements. You may feel less tired and sluggish, pain may be reduced, and you may even drop a few pounds. Start slowly with detoxes like colon cleanses, caffeine elimination, and even exercise. With others you can jump right in. Whatever you choose, your liver will thank you for your attempts. You will help protect your health for the long term and also ensure that you achieve better physical, mental, and emotional health now.

---

* Anticancer Action *

As soon as you wake up each morning, drink a big mug of warm water with lemon.

This is an important first step in daily detoxification.

It flushes your body, rehydrates you, and gives you energy to start your day

---

Chapter 8: Illnesses Linked with Cancer

In Chapter 6, we looked at the ways environmental toxins affect our health and susceptibility to developing sickness. In addition to toxins, there are illnesses and infections which may also predispose us to diseases like cancer.

For many, cancer is truly the scariest disease. It is the "C" word left unspoken, too horrific to even talk about or consider. Cancer, however, is not the only condition to be wary of or to be proactive in preventing. Did you know that there are some other illnesses which may be directly associated with cancer? They may either cause cancer or be a result of existing cancer. They may be associated with infection, chronic inflammation, or DNA mutations. They may be a result of a weakened immune system, perhaps due to cancer or autoimmune disease. This chapter is devoted to informing you of the connection between cancer and various other illnesses and to educating you about how they may be prevented.

1) Human Papilloma Virus

Human Papilloma Virus (or HPV) is considered a sexually transmitted virus, so common that it affects nearly 80% of the population. There are approximately 150 viruses in the HPV family. It is passed through skin-to-skin contact, typically affecting the genital area and/or mouth and throat regions. Some strains of HPV cause warts. These strains are typically more benign. Other less serious strains of HPV may cause no symptoms at all, and people may not ever know they carry the virus. The virus can actually also self-resolve or "shed" itself overtime. However, some high-risk HPV strains can persist and lead to cancer.

HPV can develop into cervical cancer. Among women, it is the second most common cause of cancer worldwide and the 14th most common in the USA. Cases of cervical cancer have dropped dramatically due to Pap screening tests. These tests can detect abnormal cells before they become cancerous. Doctors can remove areas of dysplasia, preventing cancer from forming. Routine Pap tests are essential, especially if one is sexually active and/or has a history of HPV.

Men are not exempt from being affected by HPV and also from being stricken with cancer due to it. Men can develop cancer of the penis. Both men and women can develop cancer of the anus, rectum, and oropharynx (cancers of the back of the throat, including the base of the tongue and tonsils). There are also reported cases in women of vaginal and vulvar cancers.

There are vaccines available that are geared to be protective from several virulent strains of the HPV virus which are known to cause cancer. One common vaccine you may have heard of is Gardasil. The vaccine can be given to both females and males from the ages of 9 through 26. Many doctors recommend vaccination before children even become sexually active in an effort to stop these harmful strains from infecting boys and girls in the future. The vaccines are not without controversy and criticism, however. Most side effects of the vaccine are the same as normal complaints after any vaccination. These are things like fainting, dizziness, nausea, fever, swelling, and redness. However, some have claimed that the HPV vaccine causes Premature Ovarian Failure (POF) or "early menopause," leading to infertility in young women. The CDC states, "[Clinical trials] found no difference in amenorrhea (when a woman of reproductive age doesn't have a period) between women who got Gardasil compared to women who received a placebo (a shot with no medicine in it). Premature ovarian failure (POF) was not found to happen among women in the Gardasil clinical trials." They go on to say that more than 80 million doses of the vaccine have been given, and only around 26 reports of ovarian failure were reported. This does not establish causation.

So, if you are a female or male under age 26 or have young children or grandchildren, should you look into administration of the HPV vaccine? Overall, studies show positive effects in preventing those virulent strains of HPV. As with any vaccine, it's a personal choice and there will always be dissidents and those in favor. Following the research is key as is discussion with your doctor.

There are other ways to avoid HPV. Use of condoms during intercourse can be very helpful. Limiting the number of sexual partners also decreases risk. Men who are circumcised are less likely to get HPV. Abstinence, of course, also prevents genital HPV. Even waiting until a later age to have sex reduces the occurrence. Getting regular Pap tests does not prevent HPV, but it can detect cancers before they begin growing.

2) Human Immunodeficiency Virus

HIV is not a thing of the past, although modern medications can make the virus essentially undetectable in the human body. In the 1980s, HIV came to the forefront. Believed to have originally been spread from chimpanzees to humans, it became the first well-known retrovirus, a group of RNA viruses that insert a DNA copy of their genome into the host cell in order to replicate. HIV was discovered to attack the immune system, destroying white blood cells (known as T-helper cells) and replicating itself instead. In the '80s, there were not many drugs to treat the disease, and for many, HIV progressed to AIDS (Acquired Immune Deficiency Syndrome). Today, people infected with HIV are much less likely to develop AIDS due to the spectacular medicine and research-based therapies available. However, if a person does develop AIDS, other conditions and illnesses can follow, ultimately leading to the person's death.

There are opportunistic infections associated with HIV/AIDS. This means that once the immune system has weakened, it can no longer fight off other infections. Some of these infections are tuberculosis, cytomegalovirus (a herpes virus), candidiasis (overall yeast infection), cryptococcal meningitis (inflammation around the brain and spinal cord), toxoplasmosis and histoplasmosis (parasites), pneumocystis (a lung infection), and cryptosporidiosis (another parasite found in the intestines). If an HIV-infected person is taking anti-retroviral drugs, antibiotics and antifungals (when needed), and staying on top of their medication regimen, their chances for developing these infections is greatly reduced.

If a person does go on to develop AIDS, there are cancers that are more likely to occur. Kaposi's sarcoma is a tumor of the blood vessel walls and appears as pink, red, or purple lesions on the skin and mouth. It can also affect internal organs. Non-Hodgkin Lymphomas are another group of cancers that can develop. Lymphoma originates in white blood cells and travels to the lymph system. Both WBCs and the lymph system are large components of one's immune system. Because HIV weakens overall immunity, it makes sense that the virus could attack the lymph system, too. HIV-positive women are also at high risk for getting cervical intraepithelial neoplasia (CIN). CIN is the growth of abnormal, pre-cancerous cells in the cervix. Over time, CIN can progress to invasive cervical cancer, in which the cancer cells grow into deeper layers of the cervix.

Prevention is key when it comes to HIV. Preventive behaviors include sexual abstinence, a monogamous relationship with an uninfected partner, consistent and correct condom use, abstinence from injection drug use, and use of sterile equipment by those needing to administer any injections. Similar precautions are recommended for those who are already HIV-positive, both to prevent infecting others and to avoid infection with other sexually transmitted and blood-borne diseases.

For those currently uninfected with HIV but who have a higher probability of acquiring the virus, there is something called "pre-exposure prophylaxis." This is a way for people who are at substantial risk of getting it to prevent HIV infection by taking a pill every day. This may apply to people who are in relationships with an HIV-infected individuals. When someone is exposed to HIV through sex or injection drug use, these medicines can work to keep the virus from establishing a permanent infection. According to the CDC, when taken consistently, pre-exposure prophylaxes have been shown to reduce the risk of HIV infection in people who are at high risk by up to 92%.

3) Hepatitis B

Hepatitis B (HBV) is a virus that infects the liver. Most cases are acute, meaning that people will acquire the disease and recover from it. However, sometimes the virus can cause chronic Hepatitis B and become a long-term illness. Over time it can damage the liver. This damage may be cirrhosis, a slowly progressing disease in which normal liver tissue is replaced with scar tissue. Or chronic Hepatitis B could cause liver cancer. Most who develop cancer have first developed cirrhosis. About 6% of liver cancers are attributed to chronic HBV.

Chronic infection with HBV is indicated by persistence of Hepatitis B surface antigen (HBsAg), a marker of active HBV infection, in the blood for more than six months. Symptoms range from nausea, vomiting, diarrhea, loss of appetite, and the tell-tale jaundice (yellowing of the skin and eyes). Infants and children affected by HBV are much more likely to develop the chronic version. In fact, the first dose of Hepatitis B vaccination is often given in the hospital immediately following birth.

HBV can be caused by contaminated injections, sexual intercourse with an infected partner, birth of a child to an infected mother, or contact with contaminated surfaces. The virus is acquired either via mucous membrane or a puncture through the skin.

Prevention of HBV can involve vaccination. Three doses are typically given for long-term immunity. As mentioned, babies are now given the vaccine over the first few months of life. Healthcare workers are typically also encouraged to get vaccinated in since they deal with bodily fluids and potential unwanted needle sticks. Also, avoiding intimate contact with infected individuals is important to avoid contracting the disease.

4) Hepatitis C

Hepatitis C (HCV) is another virus that affects the liver. This one makes up for a higher percentage of liver cancers, around 23%. Although it can cause symptoms similar to HBV, many who become infected have no immediate symptoms. It is more likely to become a chronic condition. Around 75-85% of HCV cases result in a chronic form of the disease.

The American Cancer Society states that, in the US, 60% of chronic HCV infections are attributed to injection drug use, 10% to receiving blood transfusions before donor screening, 15% to sexual transmission, 2% to healthcare workers who experience needle-stick exposures to HCV-infected patients, and 6% to infants born to HCV-infected mothers.

(About 50% of infants born to infected mothers can clear the virus without medical treatment.) Of those infected with HCV, anywhere from 5-20% will develop cirrhosis. Liver cancer can then follow.

Unlike Hepatitis B, the Hepatitis C virus does not have a vaccine. Again, prevention is key. Individuals who test positive should be provided with a medical referral, counseling, and immunizations to reduce their risk of developing severe complications and transmitting HCV to others. There are medications to treat HCV which produce sustained response rates, meaning that HCV can be undetectable in the bloodstream. The medications, however, can be quite costly.

With both HBV and HCV, alcohol should be avoided or greatly limited. Alcohol consumption sets one up for an even greater chance of developing cirrhosis.

5) Helicobacter Pylori

Helicobacter pylori (H. pylori) is a bacterial infection that colonizes in the stomach. H. pylori can be absolutely harmless with no symptoms, but it can also lead to ulcers in the stomach and small intestine as well as gastritis. Ulcers typically present as pain and burning in the stomach region. Less common ulcer symptoms include nausea, vomiting, and loss of appetite. If left untreated, ulcers can bleed and lead to anemia. Severe, prolonged cases of H. pylori infection can lead to stomach cancer or mucosal-associated-lymphoid-type (MALT) lymphoma.

H. pylori is thought to be transmitted from oral-oral routes or from fecal-oral routes. This can be due to improper washing of hands. H. pylori can also be present in contaminated food or water.

It is not an uncommon infection. The American Cancer Society reports that a study which tested blood samples over a three-year period found that 32% of adults in the U.S. had the infection. Prevalence increased steadily with increasing age, peaking at more than 50% among persons aged 50 and older.

Because H. pylori is a bacterial infection, it needs to be treated with antibiotics. Doctors usually also prescribe an acid-blocking medication to assist with efficacy of antibiotics. Blood testing, stool testing, breath testing, and endoscopy are the primary diagnostic tools.

There are some ways to avoid contracting H. pylori if it isn't already present in the body. Avoid eating poorly cooked food that might be contaminated with bacteria. Avoid unsanitary places and objects, and always wash your hands thoroughly if you do come into contact with them. The bacteria can be found in saliva, feces, vomit, and other gastric and oral secretions, so avoid touching these things or getting them into your mouth. Hand washing is critical. Unfortunately, if a loved one has the infection, you can get it by kissing them or eating from the same utensils. If a family member tests positive for H. pylori, you should also be tested.

There are some natural remedies for treating H. pylori that you could try. (However, if you are having severe symptoms or you know you are infected, you should seek medical help from your doctor.) Probiotics are a great way to introduce beneficial bacteria and assist with antibiotic treatment. Green tea is also thought to help kill or slow the growth of H. pylori. Honey has shown antibacterial abilities against the infection. Olive oil may also treat H. pylori as it remains stable in gastric acid and has been shown to be antibacterial. Licorice root is another common remedy for stomach ulcers, and it prevents H. pylori from sticking to cell walls. A compound in broccoli sprouts also shows some promise as research indicates that it reduces gastric inflammation and lowers bacterial colonization.

6) Epstein-Barr Virus

The Epstein-Barr Virus (EBV) is commonly associated with mononucleosis, or "mono" for short. It is also sometimes called the "kissing disease" because of how it's spread. The virus is found in saliva, blood, and semen. Besides intimate contact, it can be passed simply by sharing a utensil or a drinking glass with an infected person.

Many people carry the virus and never get sick. In fact, most of us have been exposed to the virus at some point in our lives. Children who get EBV often have symptoms similar to that of a cold. However, some people's infections can progress into mono. This is more common in the teenage years. Symptoms of mono include severe fatigue, fever, loss of appetite, swollen glands, sore throat, weakness, and sometimes even a rash. These symptoms can last for a couple weeks and the fatigue possibly up to several months.

Because EBV is not a bacteria, it cannot be treated with antibiotics. Mono should clear up on its own in a couple weeks. Resting and drinking plenty of fluids is the best medicine.

Prevention is key to avoiding EBV. This primarily involves avoiding close contact with anyone bearing the virus. However, symptoms often take four to six weeks before showing up. So, someone could carry the virus and be unaware.

Although most acute cases of EBV clear up within in a few days to weeks, once infected, the virus lingers in one's system. It becomes latent. In some cases, the virus may reactivate. This does not always cause symptoms, but people with weakened immune systems are more likely to develop symptoms if EBV reactivates.

The exact etiology is not known, but for some, EBV can reactivate in potentially life-threatening ways. Weakened immunity from another infection, genetics, or environmental factors are likely at fault. EBV can cause such conditions as viral meningitis, encephalitis, optic neuritis (swelling of the eye nerve), transverse myelitis (swelling of spinal cord), facial nerve and other paralysis, Guillain-Barre (an immune system disorder), multiple sclerosis, acute cerebellar ataxia (sudden uncoordinated muscle movement), sleep disorders, psychoses, pneumonia, myocarditis (swelling of the heart), and pancreatitis.

Unfortunately, EBV can also affect a person's blood and bone marrow, and lead to certain cancers. Burkitt's lymphoma was one of the first conditions found to be caused by EBV. It is a cancer of the lymphatic system. Non-Hodgkin's lymphoma and Hodgkin's disease, both also cancers of the lymphatic system, have been associated with a reoccurrence of EBV. Other cancers include nasopharyngeal (upper throat), gastric, tumors including leiomyosarcomas (of the soft tissue), and T-cell lymphomas.

Keeping one's overall immune system healthy is so important in fighting off viruses. It's hard to avoid coming into contact with EBV, and you've probably already been exposed anyway. But, protecting your immune system by eating right, avoiding toxins, getting sleep and exercise, and taking vitamins (all the tools we've mentioned in this book) will go a long way in helping you to try and prevent many of these other illnesses.

7) Diabetes

Having a diagnosis of diabetes significantly increases one's risk of developing cancer. Cancer and diabetes are diagnosed within the same individual more frequently than would be expected by chance, even after adjusting for age. This pertains primarily to Type 2 diabetes. The relative risks imparted by diabetes are greatest (about twofold or higher) for cancers of the liver, pancreas, and endometrium, and lesser (about 1.2-1.5 times higher) for cancers of the colon and rectum, breast, and bladder. Some of the other cancers associated with diabetes are kidney, thyroid, gallbladder, and chronic myeloid leukemia.

The pancreas is responsible for producing insulin. It is then transported via the portal vein to the liver. So, both the liver and the pancreas are exposed to high concentrations of endogenously produced insulin when someone has high blood sugars or is diabetic. This may be one reason for higher levels of these cancers.

Some risk factors that increase one's chance of developing diabetes also increase one's chance for developing cancer. Some risk factors are unavoidable like age, gender, and ethnicity. However, some factors are avoidable; things like being overweight, poor dietary choices, lack of physical exercise, smoking, and excessive alcohol use.

It's also thought that having diabetes may lead to cancer because of several mechanisms specific to the diabetes disease process. For one, people with diabetes have higher blood sugars. This creates an overall greater inflammatory process in the body. Remember that inflammation is a hallmark of cancer risk. Higher than normal insulin levels may also contribute. This elevated insulin can be an inherent response in the body or from exogenous injectable insulin. Remember, we previously looked at insulin-like growth factor (IGF) and its role in cancer formation.

Fortunately, Type 2 Diabetes is largely preventable. Lifestyle factors are important like reducing overall body weight, following a whole foods, unprocessed and unrefined foods diet, and exercising. Type 2 Diabetes can be reversed with these measures. And if you work to prevent diabetes, you may just prevent cancer in the process.

8) Heart Disease

Researchers have found that those who've suffered a heart attack are three times more likely to develop cancer. A survey was conducted as part of the Gallup Healthways Well-Being Index which interviewed more than 350,000 people. The relationship between heart disease and cancer was especially significant in those under 45 years of age. Researchers point out that the results do not necessarily mean that heart disease causes cancer, but they do show that cancer and chronic health conditions share many risk factors and may be interrelated. For example, cigarette smoking can increase the risk for heart disease and cancer. Likewise, obesity can cause heart disease, and cancer may also follow due to the increased inflammation associated with being overweight.

Cancer and heart disease go both ways. Some cancer treatments, including chemotherapy and radiation, can also cause heart disease or a weakening of the heart muscle called cardiomyopathy. Another heart condition, cardiac amyloidosis, is sometimes linked to multiple myeloma.

The American Heart Association suggests seven different ways to reduce your chance of getting heart disease. These prevention strategies include being physically active, controlling cholesterol, eating better, managing blood pressure, maintaining a healthy weight, reducing blood sugar, and stopping smoking.

9) Autoimmune Diseases

An autoimmune disease is a disease in which the body's immune system attacks healthy cells. The body's immune system may begin producing antibodies that instead of fighting infections, damage its own tissues. The cause of autoimmune disease is unknown. There are many theories about what triggers autoimmune diseases, including bacterial or viral infections, drugs, chemical or environmental irritants, allergens, and even food sensitivities. One may also be more susceptible to developing an autoimmune condition if a close family member has one. Underlying genetic causes are possible.

Examples of autoimmune diseases include rheumatoid arthritis, Hashimoto's thyroiditis, Graves' disease, lupus, inflammatory bowel disease (ulcerative colitis and Crohn's disease), celiac disease, multiple sclerosis, Type 1 Diabetes, Guillain-Barre syndrome, Sjogren's syndrome, Addison's disease, alopecia, psoriasis, scleroderma, myasthenia gravis, and vasculitis. And there are many more.

Some symptoms of various autoimmune conditions include but are not limited to joint and muscle pain, tremors, muscle weakness, digestive issues, weight loss, insomnia, intolerance to cold or heat, recurrent rash or hives, butterfly shaped rash across cheeks, brain fog, extreme fatigue, hair loss, dry eyes or skin, and numbness or tingling in hands or feet. Experiencing one or more of these symptoms may be reason to visit to your doctor.

If you have an autoimmune disease, your immune system can make mistakes. Your immune cells start to attack your own normal body cells. This can, unfortunately, lead to cell mutations and cancer.

Generally speaking, most people with autoimmune diseases will not develop cancer. However, some studies have reported certain types of cancer developing in people who have particular autoimmune diseases. A ten year study's review published in the journal *Anticancer Research* found multiple associations between autoimmune conditions and cancer. Researchers concluded that evidence demonstrates that chronic inflammation and autoimmunity are associated with the development of malignancy. Additionally, patients with a primary malignancy may develop autoimmune-like disease. So, again, cancer and autoimmune disease can potentially go both ways: one may cause the other.

We'll look at a few of these autoimmune/cancer connections, however there are certainly more that exist. If you have an autoimmune disease, you should do your own research and be aware of a possible connection with cancer. Keep in mind though that the risks are probably quite small.

One example is that those with celiac disease (an inability to digest gluten) are more likely to get non-Hodgkin's lymphoma, Hodgkin's disease, and small bowel cancer. When people with celiac disease eat foods containing gluten, their immune system responds by damaging the finger-like villi of the small intestine. This results in cellular damage that can lead to malignancy in the future.

Inflammatory bowel disease (IBD) can exhibit associations with gut malignancies, the primary system targeted by its inflammation. Genetic mutations in patients with IBD have been isolated and linked to an inability to rid the body of abnormal and damaged intestinal cells, subsequently causing high levels of inflammation. Patients with IBD appear to lose immune tolerance for normal gut flora. Did you know that your gut wall houses 70% of the cells that make up your immune system? An attack on the gut is an attack on immunity.

Rheumatoid arthritis (RA) is an autoimmune disease that primarily affects joints and cartilage. It creates inflammation that causes the tissue that lines the inside of joints (the synovium) to thicken, resulting in swelling and pain in and around the joints. It is a systemic disease, attacking the entire body. Cancers associated with RA include lung, kidney, thyroid, melanoma, and hematologic (blood or bone marrow) cancers.

Systemic lupus erythematosus, or lupus, is a chronic, autoimmune disease in which the body's immune system becomes hyperactive and attacks normal, healthy tissue. This results in symptoms such as inflammation, swelling, and damage to joints, skin, kidneys, blood, the heart, and lungs. Lupus makes the immune system unable to differentiate between antigens (a substance capable of inducing a specific immune response) and healthy tissue. This leads the immune system to direct antibodies against the healthy tissue. So damage can occur anywhere in the body. Cancers associated with lupus include lymphomas, breast, lung, cervical, and endometrial. It's also been found that immunosuppressive drugs given to treat lupus may increase the odds of developing cancer.

It may or may not be possible to prevent autoimmune conditions. Some theories suggest that dietary sensitivities can be at the root cause of autoimmune illnesses. Of course, for those with celiac disease, avoiding gluten is of utmost importance and can actually completely heal those with the condition.

Gluten sensitivity is also thought to trigger other autoimmune illnesses. So, one does not need to have an overt gluten allergy, but a latent sensitivity may also stimulate illness. In Chapter 3, we discussed the work of autoimmune specialist Dr. Amy Myer, M.D. She believes that everyone with autoimmune disease should avoid gluten, especially those with Hashimoto's thyroiditis. The belief is that gluten causes "leaky gut" by irritating the gut lining and making it possible for microbes, toxins, proteins, and partially digested food particles to enter into the bloodstream where they don't belong. This triggers an autoimmune response.

Unfortunately, once the gut is compromised, other foods may also cause sensitivities, so cross-reactivity may also occur. Dairy is a big culprit. Many who are sensitive to gluten are to dairy as well. Gluten is thought to trigger inflammation and also to mimic one's own body tissue. So, the body's immune system may begin to attack normal, healthy tissue instead of the foreign gluten invader.

Preventing and treating autoimmune disease (aside from traditional medications) may be one and the same. Avoiding irritating foods can be quite beneficial. In Chapter 7, we looked at some common food allergens. Doing an elimination diet, in which you avoid these foods for a period of time, can help indicate whether or not you have a sensitivity or reaction toward them. Increasing your intake of foods that heal the gut and provide good nutrition also set up your body to function optimally. These include nutrient-dense foods and foods that promote healthy gut flora like fermented foods and probiotic-rich foods. Taking quality supplements can also help ensure adequate vitamin, mineral, and micronutrient intake.

Of course, lifestyle modification is also crucial for people with autoimmune disease. This includes exercise (the right kinds, and the right amount), some sun exposure for vitamin D, stress management, sleep, and pleasure and social connection. Avoiding toxins in the environment and in your home can help. Also healing the body of any infections is crucial, be they viral, bacterial, or yeast.

10) Allergies

Having an allergic reaction causes one's immune system to enter a heightened state of activity. The interesting thing about allergies is that there is research to indicate that allergies may protect against cancer development. And, on the contrary, there is research to suggest the opposite.

Team "Allergies are Protective":

A 2011 *Time* magazine article cites a study out of Copenhagen University Hospital in Denmark which followed over 17,000 adults for over 20 years. The study found that since allergic reactions are essentially heightened immune responses to often benign compounds, such as dust or nickel or other agents, people with allergies might already be primed to attack any foreign intruders, including tumors. The study found an apparent protective effect of allergy against breast and certain skin cancers. However, the study also found that people with contact allergies were *more* likely to develop cancer of the bladder, compared with non-allergic people. It's unclear whether the bladder cancer link is due to allergen metabolites accumulating in the bladder, or whether bladder tissue is different in some way from other tissue.

A 2005 study in *Cancer Research* found that allergies and asthma were associated with a decreased risk of developing one form of brain cancer. Another 2005 study published in the *American Journal of Epidemiology* found significantly lowered risks of approximately 10% for overall cancer mortality and 20% for colorectal cancer mortality among persons with a history of both asthma and hay fever. A history of hay fever only was associated with a significantly lowered risk of pancreatic cancer mortality, and a history of asthma only was associated with a lowered risk of leukemia mortality.

In 2008, the *Quarterly Review of Biology* published a meta-analysis of 148 papers and studies that looked at the relationship between allergies and cancer. The reviewers determined that, overall, IgE antibodies (produced by the immune system) and associated allergy symptoms may serve a common protective function: the rapid expulsion of pathogens, dangerous natural toxins, and other carcinogenic antigens before they can trigger cancer in exposed tissues. The cancers most common with this inverse relationship were mouth and throat, brain glia, colon and rectum, pancreas, skin, and cervix.

For scientists who believe allergies are beneficial, the overall thought is that a hyper-stimulated immune response can actually help the body attack foreign cancer cells, just as it attacks foreign allergens.

Team "Allergies are Harmful":

A study, published in 2015 in the *Journal of Leukocyte Biology,* found just the opposite. In mice studies, inflammation was shown to raise the level of a known biomarker of cancer, which boosts the growth and spread (metastasis) of tumors. Metastasis of breast cancer to the lungs was greater in mice with pre-existing pulmonary inflammatory illnesses (like allergies or asthma). Lead researcher Vijaya L. Iragavarapu-Charyulu stated, "The research we have done is striking in that we showed pre-existing inflammation may be one of the factors that accelerates metastasis to the inflamed site." The research team went on to say that chronic inflammation, like that from chronic allergies and infections, is linked to increased risk of tumor development.

A 2004 article published in *BioMed Central Public Health* cited a study of more than 25,000 Swedish twins. The study found that allergic conditions might increase the risk of some hematological malignancies (cancers of the blood). Hives and asthma tended to increase the risk of leukemia, and childhood eczema increased the risk of non-Hodgkin's lymphoma.

Another study published in 2013 in the *American Journal of Hematology* found a connection between certain types of hematologic malignancies and allergies, but only in women. More than 60,000 participants were studied. Researchers stated, "Together, our study indicates a moderately increased risk of HMs (hematologic malignancies) in women but not men with a history of allergies to airborne allergens, especially to plant, grass, or trees." No reason was given for the difference between men and women.

What do we make of the research?

Obviously the research is conflicting and confusing. Do allergies help us fight off cancer or do they predispose us to cancer? It's clear more work needs to be done.

So, what's the take away message for you? Well, first off, don't worry if you have allergies, especially those that you cannot control. You can't avoid pollen or grass if those are allergens for you. You can try to stay away from them as much as possible, but we live on Earth and can't always control our surroundings.

However, if you can avoid allergens, you should probably do so. For example, if you know you have overt food allergies or sensitivities, of course you'll need to stay away from those. Some food allergies trigger a throat-closing, anaphylactic response, but some sensitivities may be more obscure and harder to detect. Doing food elimination diets are always a good idea to try once or twice a year to see if certain foods are causing any unwanted symptoms like headaches, migraines, digestive issues, skin issues, etc. Foods that are common culprits of sensitivities include, but are not limited to, corn, soy, gluten, dairy, eggs, nuts, and sometimes fish and shellfish.

You should visit your doctor if you have any symptoms of allergies like chronic sore throats, nasal drainage, sinus infections, eye irritation, lung irritation, skin rashes or hives, etc. Tests can be ordered to determine environmental and food allergens.

It makes sense to avoid inflammation when possible. We've talked extensively about the connection between inflammation and cancer. We've also seen that some anti-inflammatory foods prevent cancer and some anti-inflammatory meds like aspirin may also help to prevent the disease.

If the research showing allergies prevent cancer is correct, you may be in luck! Your body may be primed to fight off tumors better than people who don't have allergies. However, it's probably still best to avoid allergens overall when possible. Doing so simply helps wards off inflammation, not to mention the nuisance allergies cause.

Final Thoughts on Illnesses Linked with Cancer

Many illnesses can be prevented. Others may be genetic or may be caused by unknown factors. The reality is we are not God. We can take preventative steps to lessen our chances of contracting viruses or cancer. We can be on top of the latest research, have our diets completely in check, sleep well, and exercise adequately, and yet, cancer and disease still plague our society. That doesn't mean we shouldn't try to prevent it, however. Our health really is more in our hands than we may believe. Because our bodies are our temples and we only get one, we need to take care of them *every* day. By following the preventative tips in this chapter and throughout the book, you'll be ahead of the game. Above all, always focus on the positive in your life and all that you're grateful for. We don't want to focus our energy worrying about getting sick. Living positively does so much more for our health and well-being.

---

* Anticancer Action *

If you are sexually active and not in a monogamous relationship, always use a condom to prevent the spread of sexually transmitted diseases and viruses like Hepatitis B & C.

Keep your immunity up by eating **10** servings of fruit and vegetables per day.

(Some tips to get it all in: Make a breakfast smoothie with various fruits and spinach. Eat a big salad for lunch topped with tomatoes, carrots, broccoli, and berries. Snack on apples or pears. Eat a side salad and/or steamed vegetables with your dinner.)

Chapter 9: Lifestyle Practices to Incorporate

Now we can get to the fun stuff! Creating a healthy body doesn't have to be all about restriction. We can incorporate lifestyle practices that make us feel good, energetic, and not at all deprived. According to the American Cancer Society, only 5-10% of cancers are directly related to genes. This is great news! **That means that up to 90-95% of cancer can be avoided.** The lifestyle choices we make, the foods we eat, and the amount of exercise we incorporate into our daily lives can have an important impact on our overall risk.

Earlier we looked at all of the wonderfully nourishing and delicious foods we can eat to optimize our nutrition. If you missed it, please review Chapter 2 for a comprehensive list of those foods. Finding new recipes or checking out restaurants that provide dishes with anti-inflammatory, anti-angiogenic foods can be a really fun experience. You *can* treat yourself and still be very healthy.

There are lots of other ways beyond diet to also encourage optimal health. Sometimes health must start in the brain. Being positive, optimistic, and feeling loved are often just as important to our well-being as eating well and exercising. We'll take a look at some important lifestyle practices that can easily fit into our schedules and that will go a long way in boosting our immunity.

1) Exercise

Have you heard that "sitting is the new smoking"? A study published in the *Journal of the National Cancer Institute,* which looked at more than four million people and over 60,000 cancer cases, found that sitting for long periods of time increases your risk for colon, endometrial, and possibly lung cancer. The study found that even in physically active individuals, sitting increased the risk of developing cancer, and continued to increase with each two-hour segment of sitting time.

Exercise is important in the fight against cancer for various reasons. More than two dozen studies have shown that women who exercise have a 30-40% lower risk of breast cancer than their sedentary peers. Exercise lowers estrogen, so frequent exercisers have less risk for estrogenic cancers. Also, more than three dozen studies show exercisers reduce their risk of colon cancer by 20% or more compared to sedentary people, and the benefits are seen in both men and women. These are just a few examples of how exercise statistically reduces cancer risk.

Besides just lowering estrogen levels, exercise can decrease blood sugar and insulin levels. It also improves circulation and increases lymphatic drainage. It's also been suggested that apoptosis is triggered by exercise, causing cancer cells to die.

Even though we know it's good for us, exercise can seem like such a daunting and unpleasant task, especially for those who have never exercised. But, I'm here to tell you, it can be very easy to incorporate and does not have to be a grueling chore. A few minutes of exercise daily or several times a week is all it takes to decrease your risk for cancer and other diseases.

It's a common myth that "more is better." When it comes to exercise, this is just simply not true. In fact, endurance athletes are actually more prone to injuries and other serious conditions. Overuse injuries like stress fractures, plantar fasciitis, tendonitis, and knee and hip pain are common. Other serious consequences can also be attributed to endurance training, conditions like exercise-induced asthma, hyponatremia (low sodium levels), and cardiac damage from chronic and repetitive over-taxing of the heart. If you enjoy endurance training like running marathons or doing IRONMAN triathlons, then train wisely, listen to your body, and continue to enjoy that. However, if you're like most of the population who prefer less extreme measures for fitness, you can be just as healthy if not healthier by doing simpler and less time-consuming exercise.

The general consensus is that 30 minutes of exercise a day is a great goal. Experts recommend a combination of walking (or other cardiovascular exercise) and strength training. Cardiovascular exercise improves circulation and the ability to rid the body of toxins. A study published in 2016 in *JAMA Internal Medicine* reviewed 12 studies that took place over 17 years. More than 1.4 million participants with an average age of 59 were studied. After compiling all the evidence, researchers found that the risk of developing seven cancer types was more than 20% lower among the most active participants as compared with the least active. Interesting and important to note, researchers also found that people with lower activity levels, those who do two and a half hours a week of brisk walking (averaging only 13 minutes a day), still had notably lower cancer risk, even if it was not quite as low as those who did more activity.

Strength training also has links to increased cancer prevention. A study published in the journal *Cancer Epidemiology, Biomarkers and Prevention* tracked the lifestyles of over 8,500 men for more than two decades. Each volunteer had regular medical check-ups that included tests of their muscular strength. The men who regularly worked out with weights and had the highest muscle strength were between 30-40% less likely to lose their life to a deadly tumor.

Another great option is high-intensity interval training, or HIIT for short. HIIT is a training technique in which you give all-out effort for intense bursts of exercise, followed by short, sometimes active, recovery periods. This type of training gets and keeps your heart rate up and burns more fat in less time. It can increase your endurance and cardiac output and rev your metabolism, too. A 2006 study published in the *Journal of Physiology* found that after eight weeks of doing HIIT workouts, subjects could bicycle twice as long as they could before the study, while maintaining the same pace.

The great news about HIIT is that it only takes about 15 minutes three times a week to get results. Examples of HIIT exercise might be running as fast as you can for one minute and then walking for two minutes, repeating this pattern five times. Or you could do walking weighted lunges interspersed with crunches. There are also a myriad of HIIT videos on

YouTube. You can modify them to an appropriate level for yourself. So, if you can't run, maybe you can do jumping jacks or toe touches. You get the idea.

So, just do what you can to "move." Getting up from your desk or couch to walk around every 20 minutes or so will go a long way in keeping you healthier. Aim to try to exercise a few times a week. Maybe try to go for a walk after dinner most evenings. You can always work your way to longer, more frequent, and/or more intense workouts. But start slowly. It's best not to begin too forcefully so as to avoid burn-out or injury. Above all, find something you like to do. Nothing is worse than performing an exercise that is boring or feels wrong to you. There are many options besides walking, running, HIIT, and strength-training. You can try Zumba, swimming, water aerobics, yoga, Pilates, dancing, skiing, cycling, adult kickball or other fun league activities, etc. Experiment and find something you enjoy. Exercise can be a great stress relief and past-time. You can even meet some great friends along the way.

2) Maintain Friendships

Having a rewarding social life goes a long way in improving your health and overall well-being. "Researchers have found that having even *one* close friend that you confide in can extend your life by as much as 10 years," says sociologist and relationship coach Jan Yager, PhD, author of *Friendshifts*. Yager also states, "Numerous studies also show that recovery from a major health challenge, such as a heart attack or cancer, is enhanced because of friendship."

A 2000 study published in *Psychological Review* found that when women gather around other women or around children, they release oxytocin and other hormones. Oxytocin has been called the "love hormone" or "cuddle hormone" because it is released during intimate contact like breastfeeding or at the beginning of a new love relationship. Oxytocin, in conjunction with other female hormones, promotes a pattern of what researchers call "tend and befriend" instead of "fight or flight." This combination is a de-stressor and helps promote relaxation and a calming effect. This helps improve overall health. If you're female, having close friends or being in close relationship with children is beneficial for your wellness.

Men also benefit from having friendships. An Australian study followed male and female seniors for over a decade. The study found that those who had close friendships, above and beyond that of family, outlived those with fewer friends by 22%.

A meta-analysis of 148 studies on friendships was performed through Brigham Young University in 2010. Researchers concluded that the influence of social relationships on risk for mortality is comparable with other significant risk factors (like physical health or active lifestyles). Having social relations improved life span by as much as 50% in some instances. Studies that took into account more than one aspect of a person's relationship (for instance, social network size and how integrated a person is with that network) were better predictors of mortality.

Why are friendships so beneficial? Besides those "feel good" hormones that can be released, friends help us deal with stress. Having someone to talk to and being able to vent frustrations is good for us. Friends can encourage us to be healthy. Maybe we get out of the house more often; maybe we exercise with them; maybe we visit doctors on the advice of our friends; and maybe we just become more positive when we can laugh with someone.

Sometimes, it's hard to meet others. Perhaps you've moved to a new area. Maybe you've just had a baby and are looking for other "mom friends." There are a plethora of community groups, so check with your town or city's webpage. Churches and libraries often have groups or social gatherings. There are also sites like www.meetup.com (which also has an app) that offer a variety of ways to connect with others who share similar interests. It just takes a little exploration.

Although it doesn't replace one-on-one interactions, social media can also give us a boost. Even if you're home-bound or don't have a lot of close friends, having acquaintances on Facebook, for example, can improve your mood and make you feel a part of a larger community.

3) Have a Positive Outlook and Be Grateful

Seeing the glass as "half-full" may not only improve your mood, it may prolong your life. According to the Mayo Clinic, optimism is an effective part of stress management and provides health benefits. Researchers have found that people who are more positive have an increased life span, lower rates of depression, greater resistance to colds and viruses, better cardiovascular health, and better coping skills.

A study published in September 2013 in a journal of the *American Heart Association* looked at 607 patients in a hospital in Denmark. It found that patients whose moods were more positive were 58% more likely to live at least another five years. Another study in Norway found that people with a strong sense of humor outlived those who don't laugh as much. The difference was particularly notable for those battling cancer.

Understandably, being positive is easier said than done. Some people seem to be inherently more optimistic. Others may have been dealt more hardships in their lives and find being positive almost impossible. But there are ways to work on being more positive in your daily life.

For one, turn on a funny television show, YouTube channel, or movie. It's true that laughter is the best medicine. A recent study out of Washington University in St. Louis found for the first time that laughing gas (nitrous oxide) shows promise for helping symptoms of treatment-resistant depression. Providing ourselves with opportunities for laughter can be a great mood booster with lasting effects. Laughter also relaxes your body, improves your immunity by decreasing stress hormones and increasing infection-fighting antibodies, boosts endorphins, decreases pain, increases blood flow, and burns calories. A University of Kansas study found that smiling—even fake smiling—reduces heart rate and blood pressure during stressful situations. So even if you're not feeling so happy, faking it can actually elevate your mood!

Another way to achieve an optimistic outlook is to simply practice gratitude. When we are grateful, we can't be angry and resentful at the same time. One recent study from the University of California San Diego's School of Medicine found that people who were more grateful actually had better heart health, specifically less inflammation and healthier heart rhythms. "Clinical trials indicate that the practice of gratitude can have dramatic and lasting effects in a person's life," said Robert A. Emmons, professor of psychology at UC Davis. "It can lower blood pressure, improve immune function and facilitate more efficient sleep." You can start by keeping a gratitude journal. Gratitude journals can be as simple as writing down three things you're grateful for each day. There are even apps for your phone that allow you to track your daily entries. Being grateful reduces our stress hormones, has a calming effect, and helps us to focus on all that is good.

Even those who already have a cancer diagnosis can greatly benefit from positive vibes and gratitude. A recent study shows that people with more flexible and optimistic outlooks have better coping strategies that help facilitate cancer treatment and recovery.

So, even if you feel like you're actually a "glass half-empty" kind of person, remember that there are ways to change that mindset to improve your health. Start with being kind to yourself and practicing forgiveness. You can begin each day with affirmations, positive statements that uplift you, renew your sense of purpose, and keep you grounded. Affirmations are phrases like, "I will be a blessing to everyone I meet today," or "I am in charge of how I feel, and today I am choosing happiness." If you're a

Pinterest fan, you can find some beautiful affirmations there. Or simply Google "affirmations," and you'll find some good ones. Follow your daily affirmations with a few quick entries in your gratitude journal. These can be as simple as "I am grateful for my family, for the sunshine, and for my health." This sets the stage for positive thoughts and reminds us of people and things that are meaningful to us. Then, smile and laugh often, even if you don't feel like it. Doing these physical activities can trick your brain into believing you are happier by releasing feel-good hormones that actually do make you feel happier and more optimistic. Finally, hug someone. Even if it's your cat or dog. Hugging (or other close physical contact) releases oxytocin, resulting in lowered cortisol and stress hormones and increased feelings of calmness and happiness.

4) Find Stress Relief

Stress is an inevitable part of life. We all have it. But how we deal with it is of utmost importance. Do you let stress kick you to the curb, or do you approach stress with battle armor? When we have battle armor, tactics that enable us to cope with and tackle stress, we can more readily rise from the ashes unscathed ... or at least only mildly bruised. Some of these coping mechanisms can also be rewarding and bring much needed relaxation.

When we talk about stress, we're really talking about increased stress hormones (like cortisol, adrenaline, and norepinephrine) and their effects on the body. Some stress is acute, like the stress you experience when you are in a car accident. Some stress is chronic, like the stress from your work which accumulates over time.

Adrenaline is that "fight or flight" hormone which comes to us in the face of immediate stress or in a dangerous situation. It gets your heart rate pumping. Norepinephrine is similar to adrenaline in that it is released during acute stress. It makes you hyper-aware and alert, ready to take action. Then, we have cortisol. Cortisol takes longer to be released, but it also remains elevated much longer. When you live in a state of prolonged, chronic stress (like when you have a stressful family life for example), cortisol takes over. It helps to regulate changes that occur in the body as result of prolonged stress. It modulates things like blood sugar, immune responses, blood pressure, nervous system activity, and anti-inflammatory actions. The problem is, chronic elevated cortisol is not good for the body. Too much cortisol can suppress the immune system, increase blood pressure and sugar, decrease libido, produce acne, contribute to obesity, and more. Essentially, after a while, cortisol and stress are not our friends, and they can lead us into chronic illness or disease as well.

So how do we work to decrease cortisol and other stress hormones? As we just saw, hugging and physical touch are important for reducing stress. Being connected in this way with others makes us feel calmer and loved. We feel more equipped to cope with stressful situations when we have others to both lean on and rely on.

Finding ways to relax is also critical. What calms and relaxes you? Of course we'd all love to lie on a beach in the sunshine and listen to the waves. But how many of us can actually do that regularly? We need to find ways to incorporate relaxation into our everyday routines.

Restorative exercises like yoga encourage you to focus on the movements and moment at hand. Being present and attentive helps curtail the stresses of the day. Yoga also involves deep breathing which floods the body with oxygen, promotes blood flow, and reduces stress and blood pressure. Cardiovascular exercise can provide stress relief, too. Although it is not inherently calming, activities like running can increase endorphins which help to wash away stress and provide us with a clearer mind.

Epsom salt baths are another relaxing ritual. Epsom salt is not actually salt but a naturally occurring pure mineral compound of magnesium and sulfate. Studies have shown that magnesium and sulfate are both readily absorbed through the skin. Magnesium plays a number of roles in the body including reducing inflammation, helping muscle and nerve function, and helping to prevent artery hardening. It helps with the production of serotonin, that feel-good chemical that eases tension. Sulfates help improve the absorption of nutrients, flush toxins, and help ease migraine headaches. Epsom salt baths help to reduce stress, relax the body, and ease pain and muscle aches. Interestingly, they also help to detoxify the body by pulling out unwanted toxins through reverse osmosis. Who wouldn't love a nice hot soak after a long day?

Listening to music can also be a great stress relief. Playing calm music has a positive effect on the brain and body, can lower blood pressure, and reduce cortisol. Research has shown that music can bring order and security to disabled and distressed children. It can reduce stress and anxiety in hospitalized patients. It can reduce the sensation of chronic pain. It can relieve depression and elevate moods. And it also boosts quality of life among adult cancer patients.

Talking to a friend, loved one, or counselor can go a long way. It actually *is* good to vent sometimes. It's also good to let out emotions. Crying, laughing, or even expressing anger through our words helps us release pent up emotions that may be weighing us down. When we can talk through our days and stressful events, we take on a sense of ownership and an ability to reflect. We can be on top of the stress instead of letting it take over our lives. We may find new perspectives on how to deal with stressful events. It's also important just to know we are not alone. Writing down our feelings is another useful strategy. Bringing our thoughts to the surface helps us reflect and find out what is causing stress. After we know, we can find better ways to cope.

Meditation and prayer can also be quite useful in relieving stress. Research suggests that daily meditation may alter the brain's neural pathways, making you more resilient to stress. Mindfulness is a concept reaching back to the teachings of Buddha. It involves bringing all of one's attention to internal experiences occurring in the present moment, practicing intentional, nonjudgmental awareness. Prayer provides that inner sense of well-being and allows us to turn our concerns over to a higher power. During times of prayer and meditation, we also quiet our minds and eliminate the outside chaos to focus our thoughts and breaths. Best of all, science has linked meditation and contemplative prayer to cancer reduction because practicing them is said to lengthen our telomeres. Telomeres protect our chromosomes and healthy cells and also hep to ward off abnormal cancer cells. Shortened telomeres are associated with aging, cancer risk, and premature death.

5) Practice Spirituality

Dr. Roberta Lee, integrative medicine specialist and author of *The SuperStress Solution*, states, "Research shows that people who are more religious or spiritual use their spirituality to cope with life. They're better able to cope with stress, they heal faster from illness, and they experience increased benefits to their health and wellbeing."

While prayer is quite healing, belonging to a church or other religious organization has its benefits, too. Being a part of a larger, faith-based community gives one a sense of fellowship.

A study conducted in North Carolina found that frequent churchgoers had larger social networks and more contact with, more affection for, and more kinds of support from those people than their unchurched counterparts. We know that social support is directly tied to better health.

According to a 2016 study from Harvard T.H. Chan School of Public Health, women who attended religious services more than once per week were more than 30% less likely to die during a 16-year follow-up than women who never attended. Those who attended weekly had 26% lower risk. The data came from the famous Nurses' Health Study which followed over 70,000 women for 20 years. The study also found that women who attended religious services once per week or more had a decreased risk of cardiovascular mortality (27%) and cancer mortality (21%). "Our results suggest that there may be something important about religious service attendance beyond solitary spirituality," said Tyler Vanderweele, professor of epidemiology at Harvard Chan School and author of the study. "Part of the benefit seems to be that attending religious services increases social support, discourages smoking, decreases depression, and helps people develop a more optimistic or hopeful outlook on life."

The study looked at mostly those who attended Protestant or Catholic churches. However, being a part of any larger faith-based community has the same benefits. You may go to a synagogue, mosque, prayer-group, Bible study, or even just get together with like-minded individuals who encourage your faith or spiritual journey.

Beyond the fellowship of church, embracing our spirituality and/or practicing religion connects us with a higher power. Accepting that not everything is in our control alleviates some of the stress we place upon ourselves. When we can turn to God or a higher power in prayer, and when we read scriptures, we focus on something other than ourselves and gain insight which can help transform our lives.

6) Sleep

Sleep plays a vital role in your health during your whole lifetime. Babies and teenagers are not the only ones who need good quality sleep. We all do! Getting enough quality sleep at the right times can help protect your mental health, physical health, quality of life, and safety. A lack of sleep is associated with lower moods, obesity, and a myriad of illnesses. Although it may seem difficult to do, we all need to carve out more time for sleep. It is essential to our health, perhaps even more important than exercising and eating well.

For many, there never seem to be enough hours in the day. We're a busy society. Between work, kids, extracurricular activities, community events, social calendars, and busy home lives, we are always on the go. We try to jam too much into our schedules and leave little time for relaxation and rest. We may be accomplishing a lot, but boy are we tired! Productivity can actually become counterproductive when it comes to our health.

Our emotional health is something we don't always associate with sleep, but it plays a huge part in our daily attitude and energy. While you're sleeping, your brain is preparing for the next day. Studies show that sleep helps us remember things and improves learning, which is why it is so important for school-age children. Sleep helps us make decisions, control our emotions, and cope with life's changes. Sleep deficiency is linked with depression, mood swings, and even suicide.

When you function on little sleep, your reaction times also slow considerably. This is when accidents are more likely to occur. We've all heard of sleepy drivers who crash their cars because they simply couldn't keep their eyes open. According to the National Sleep Foundation's 2005 *Sleep in America* poll, 60% of adult drivers –- about 168 million people –- say they have driven a vehicle while feeling drowsy. More than one-third, 37% or 103 million people, have actually fallen asleep at the wheel! In fact, of those who have nodded off, 4% or approximately 11 million drivers, admit they have had an accident or near accident because they dozed off or were too tired to drive safely.

Of course, it isn't only just dangerous to drive a car when sleepy, it can also be hazardous to work and/or make decisions. Fatigue worsens your hand-eye coordination and makes it harder for you to communicate. Your brain does not process information or solve problems as well as it should. You also tend to take more risks. This means that your chance of making errors goes up. If you work in an environment that involves physical labor, you could be at risk for injury. Even if you don't work in such an environment, you could make mistakes that could cost your company money, that could threaten work relationships, and certainly that could make you not enjoy your job.

As far as illness goes, adequate sleep can help you prevent sickness and disease. When you're sleeping, your immune system produces protective cytokines and infection-fighting antibodies and cells. It uses these tools to fight off foreign substances like bacteria and viruses. Studies have shown that lack of sleep or sleep disturbances are associated with higher rates of breast, prostate, and colorectal cancers. In addition, research suggests that people who have sleep apnea have an increased risk of developing any type of cancer.

Those who work the night shift are also at greater risk of developing certain cancers. In 2007, the *International Agency for Research on Cancer* declared "shift work that involves circadian disruption is probably carcinogenic to humans." The evidence is strongest for breast cancer, although the risk of prostate and colorectal cancer may also be increased by shift work. Possible reasons for increases in cancer are that working at night, and the accompanying light, reduces the body's production of melatonin which has direct and indirect anticancer effects. Melatonin is actually a powerful antioxidant.

Sleep disruption stimulates the brain to release glucocorticoids, which results in depression of immune function. There is probably a decreased production of vitamin D, a cancer-preventing vitamin, due to lack of direct exposure to sunshine. A disruption in circadian rhythms is also thought to result in changes in the control of cell and tissue proliferation.

Some researchers suggest dimming computer screens and/or wearing blue light-blocking glasses at night. These actually look like orange-lensed sunglasses. In a study by scientists at Quebec's Universite Laval, nightshift workers used blue-light blocking glasses at or near the end of their overnight shifts for four weeks. At the end of study period, their overall sleep amounts increased, as did their sleep efficiency. This may be one way to avoid the harmful consequences of shift work.

Blue light is actually harmful for the rest of us, too. At the end of a busy day, so often we're drawn to the vegging out in front of the TV, computers, or our phones. However, the blue and white light emitted from these devices is counterproductive to our good sleep. They prevent our brains from releasing melatonin, a hormone that tells our bodies it's nighttime.

In a 2016 study, nearly 850 Flemish adults found that using a mobile phone after turning the lights off was associated with worse sleep quality, more insomnia, and more symptoms of fatigue. If you must watch TV or use your phone at night, try to turn off all devices an hour before you aim to fall asleep. You can also use a filter that blocks blue light. The newer iPhones also have settings which dim your screen with a yellowish glow for night-time use. You may want to purchase some cool, orange sunglasses, too! Wearing these a couple hours before bedtime can counteract the light emitted from any device.

What are other ways we can relax and get some good quality sleep? The Epsom salts baths we mentioned above are also tremendous ways to relax. They allow for a warm soak which effectively raises our body temperature, and the subsequent drop helps with our sleep. Epsom salts also allow magnesium, the relaxation mineral, to enter your bloodstream and promote sleep. Try taking an Epsom salt bath a half hour before bedtime.

Taking a magnesium supplement in the evening can also help promote sleep. In Chapter 4, we learned that the majority of the population is deficient in magnesium, so taking a supplement can be beneficial for various reasons. Start by taking 400 mg. If you don't see results, you can work your way up to 600 mg or even 800 mg. It can truly help you sleep like a baby.

Another supplement that many regard as useful is melatonin. There are mixed reviews on melatonin, however, because of its potential addictive properties. Once people take it regularly, sometimes they are unable to fall asleep without it. It's also technically a hormone that our bodies produce, but the melatonin on shelves is synthetic and is unregulated by the FDA. It's possible to take more than you need as well. This can result in next day drowsiness. If you do take melatonin, be sure to only take it when necessary and always take the lowest possible dose first. Some people swear by its effectiveness, though. Other supplements to consider could be valerian root, GABA, or the amino acid L-theanine. These may provide some promising help.

As far as other sleep aids go, I do not recommend prescription drugs like Ambien. This is just a personal choice, but I'll explain why. They absolutely do work to induce sleep. However, having been in the medical field and having administered these drugs to patients, I've witnessed some pretty scary side effects. Often, people fall asleep quite quickly after taking the medication. However, sometimes after two or three hours, they may wake up in a very dazed and confused state. They are not aware of their surroundings and may do dangerous things or act in atypical ways. While working at a hospital, I cared for a woman who was prescribed a sleeping aid. Approximately two hours after she took the medicine, she awoke and tried to go to the restroom. The problem was, she hadn't walked without a walker or other assistive device in months. Despite having a walker nearby as well as a bedside commode, she attempted to walk unassisted to the bathroom. She simply was not of full mental capacity, being groggy and heavily sedated. She fell and broke her hip. After being fully awakened, she remembered none of it, only that she now was in excruciating pain.

Do you remember the news story of Kerry Kennedy, daughter of Robert Kennedy, who crashed her car after taking Ambien? In her testimony, she claimed that the drug "overtook" her. There have been a number of driving accidents linked with such medications. If you do take a prescription sleeping aid, work closely with your doctor. Know the side effects. Only take the amount prescribed or even less than that. Always be careful, and always take it immediately before bed.

Besides taking supplements or medications, you can use some other tried and true methods. Try to sleep in a completely dark room. This helps produce the naturally occurring hormone, melatonin. Use black-out curtains and blinds. Also try to avoid having light-emitting clocks or other electronics nearby. You might also want to purchase a sleeping mask. My husband loves his lavender-scented, black silk sleeping mask.

By the way, lavender is a calming herb and essential oil and has actually been studied and deemed effective for sleep. It can be diffused into the air via an essential-oil diffuser. This can also add some moisture to the air. Alternatively, you could try just putting a few drops of lavender oil on a tissue and tucking it under your pillow.

The temperature of your bedroom makes a huge difference as well. In general, the suggested bedroom temperature should be between 60 and 67 degrees Fahrenheit for optimal sleep. Dr. Rachel Salas, MD, a neurologist at Johns Hopkins University who specializes in sleep medicine, cites a National Sleep Foundation study that puts the magic number at 65 degrees. Your body's core temperature is naturally low during deep sleep. It starts to raise towards the end of your sleep cycle, as a sort of signal to your body that it's time to wake up. If your room is too warm, this can create restlessness or insomnia, both of which interfere with appropriate sleep cycles and melatonin production.

You probably know other tips to get a better night's sleep, but let's look at some anyway. Cut the caffeine early. If you're sensitive to it, you should try to avoid any caffeine after 2:00 PM. It can interfere with circadian rhythms. Aim to be in bed around 10:00 PM if possible. Scientists believe that the best time to go to bed is between 10:00 PM and 11:00 PM. This is because your body temperature starts to drop between these times, as does your body's cortisol level. And as darkness approaches, your brain begins to release melatonin. If you do go to bed at a decent time but you can't sleep, get up. Be sure to do something relaxing like reading a book under dim light. However, staying in bed when your body is not ready for sleep can be counterproductive and can create stress for you. Try some progressive muscle relaxation, gentle yoga, meditate, and/or pray. Relaxing your body and mind are the keys to quality sleep.

7) Have Sex

Best news ever! Yes, having sex can increase your immunity and decrease your chances of developing some cancers. Researchers at Wilkes University in Pennsylvania found that college students who had sex once or twice a week had higher levels of a certain antibody compared to students who had sex less often. Sexually active people take fewer sick days overall.

A study published in *JAMA* also found that frequent ejaculation (we're talking 21+ times a month!) in middle-aged or older (50+) men decreased disease risk of prostate cancer. As for women, research has found that menopausal women who had sex every week had estrogen levels twice as high as their abstaining counterparts. This is significant because during menopause, estrogen levels drop dramatically which can cause a host of other problems like hot flashes, mood swings, memory issues, increased cardiovascular issues, osteoporosis, incontinence, etc. Also, orgasms release a large amount of oxytocin into the bloodstream. This is great news, not only for the feel good factor but because oxytocin can decrease breast cancer risk in women.

Other health benefits of sex include lowering blood pressure, lowering heart attack risk, decreasing pain, and improving sleep. Of course, sex is a huge stress reliever, so you reap the benefits of that as well.

What if you don't have a sexual partner? Self-stimulation can be just as helpful in releasing oxytocin and reaping the benefits of orgasm. Also, just cuddling with someone works. Hugging releases oxytocin as well. Just a 10-second hug a day can boost your immune system, fight off infections, lower depression rates, and reduce stress.

8) Breastfeed

Breastfeeding lowers the risk of breast cancer, especially in premenopausal women. According to Rachel King, a health education specialist in MD Anderson's Cancer Prevention Center, breastfeeding longer than the recommended six months can provide additional protection. A meta-analysis of 47 different studies found that women who breastfed for a lifetime total of more than two years (for all of their children combined) got the most benefit.

Most women who breastfeed experience hormonal changes during lactation that delay their menstrual periods. This reduces a woman's lifetime exposure to hormones like estrogen, which can promote breast cancer cell growth. Women's risk for ovarian cancer also diminishes since ovulation is typically prevented during lactation.

Nursing is obviously also beneficial for babies. Breastfeeding helps strengthen a child's immune system. Antibodies pass from mother's milk to her child. This helps lower the child's risks of ear infections, as well as respiratory and digestive problems. Research also shows that children who were breastfed tend to have lower rates of obesity, even later in life. A 2015 meta-analysis of 18 studies published in *JAMA Pediatrics* found that breastfeeding a child for six months or longer was associated with a 19% lower risk for childhood leukemia, compared to children who had been breastfed for less time or not at all. Another of their analyses revealed that children who are ever breastfed, compared to those who were never breastfed, had an 11% lower risk for childhood leukemia.

Not every mother is able to breastfeed. Sometimes anatomical issues in either the mother or baby make it impossible. Sometimes babies just have difficulty latching. Sometimes mothers suffer from severe postpartum depression and simply cannot. Sometimes it's just a personal choice not to breastfeed. If a mother is having difficulty but still wants to try, lactation consultants or the La Leche League may be of great service. However, even with all of the assistance in the world, sometimes it's just not possible.

If a woman cannot breastfeed or has never had biological children, it truly is not the end of the world. There are plenty of other ways to prevent cancer in the mother through lifestyle, diet, and exercise. Babies also thrive just fine on formula. So, a mother should not be ashamed or made to feel guilty for not nursing.

9) Lose Weight

I know, I know ... easier said than done. Losing weight is the bane of Americans' existence. Every New Year's Eve rolls around, and millions of us make resolutions to lose weight and get healthier. We join gyms, and go for a couple months. We enroll in popular diet and weight loss support groups, and follow the plans for a couple months. We go to the store and stock our refrigerator and pantry with healthy foods and toss out the junk.

This, too, lasts a couple months. Then what happens? We fall back into the daily grind. Stress overwhelms us again, and we reach for comfort foods. We don't like to feel hungry. It's too much work. We don't have time for the gym. We gain back the few pounds we lost, and this makes us feel defeated. So goes the vicious cycle of depression, overeating, and subsequent weight loss attempts.

It's not entirely our fault. Today's convenience food is hyper-palatable. Food manufacturers have found ways to add sugar, salt, oils, and flavoring in just the right amounts to make our food so tasty, we literally cannot stop overeating. It turns on brain chemicals, those endogenous opioids, which make us feel so darn good while we're eating. This is a huge reason why it's so important to stay away from the junk food and most bagged or boxed items. They are making us fat.

Obesity is linked with many health issues including cancer. According to the National Cancer Institute, obesity increases a person's inflammation which can, over time, cause DNA damage that leads to cancer. Fat tissue also produces excess estrogen which is associated with breast, endometrial, ovarian, and some other cancers. Obese people often have increased blood levels of insulin and insulin-like growth factor-1 (IGF-1) which is associated with increased cancer risk. The NIH also cites a study from the GLOBOCAN project that estimated that, in 2012 in the United States, about 28,000 new cases of cancer in men (3.5%) and 72,000 in women (9.5%) were due to being overweight or obese.

So, what should we do? We know that exercise is good for us, but over-exercising is not. "Calories in vs. calories out" is not actually entirely true. Sure, we can't pig out every day and hope to lose weight. But not all calories are created equal. When we consume high carb and/or high sugar foods, especially of the refined version, our blood sugar and insulin spike. And if these foods are also devoid of any micronutrients, our bodies essentially feel as those we haven't eaten ... because we really haven't eaten "food." We've eaten synthetic, processed, calorie-laden junk. We are left wanting more.

However, if we eat nutrient dense foods, filled with natural fibers, protein, and fat, we are satiated and really don't desire more. We're talking vegetables, fruits, protein from meat, and fats like avocado, olives/olive oil, and coconut oil. If you reread Chapter 2, you'll learn about the foods that our bodies really need and innately crave. Foods that also can prevent cancer and disease.

In my opinion, following a diet closest to what our ancestors consumed will not only help to restore health but will help with weight loss as well. Paleo diets have become a fad, it seems, however there is a lot of merit in following such a lifestyle. Paleo-compliant foods consist largely of fruits, vegetables, meat and fish, organ meat, eggs, bone broth, tubers (like sweet potatoes and sometimes regular white potatoes), nuts and seeds, herbs and spices, and fats (avocado, coconut oil, olives, and olive oil). Foods to avoid are processed foods, sugar, soft drinks, grains, most dairy products, legumes, artificial sweeteners, vegetable oils, margarine, and trans fats. This may seem daunting, but these are just general guidelines as there are variations to the diet. Some Paleo followers add butter and ghee (a type of clarified butter) or even full fat, grass-fed yogurt or dairy. Some believe Stevia is fine to use as a sweetener. Honey and maple syrup can be used in small amounts. Some add white rice (less allergenic) or quinoa (actually a seed), but gluten is always avoided. Eggs and/or nuts are also avoided by those who are sensitive or have reactions.

Overall, the Paleo diet works to eliminate possible food allergens and toxic foods, creating a less inflamed body. If you choose to follow this lifestyle, you'll quickly find that certain foods you'd previously eaten may have been causing those headaches, tummy issues, skin conditions, or a host of other aches and ailments you'd been experiencing. The Paleo diet may benefit people who want to prevent cancer and patients undergoing treatment because of less glucose in the blood, lower insulin levels, better insulin response, less inflammation and more cancer-fighting micronutrients.

Of course, the Paleo way is only one approach as far as weight loss diets go. There are a myriad of diet plans on the market, some that require subscriptions and/or weigh-ins. Others you may find online for free. Some require calorie counting. Others prohibit certain foods or food groups. It's your choice which diet you may follow, but try to find one that is sustainable in the long run. If you're drastically limiting calories and cutting out too many foods, you may end up bingeing and feel deprived. Also, strict low-calorie diets usually are not maintainable long-term. Find a way that nourishes your body with nutrient-dense foods and allows you to feel satisfied so that your health is not jeopardized for the sake of slimness.

Previously, we looked at some ways to detoxify your body. Detoxing can help us eliminate harmful toxins from food or other sources that literally weigh us down. You may find some of those ideas helpful for weight loss as well.

Final Thoughts on Lifestyle Practices to Incorporate

Being healthy can be quite fun and rewarding. Making time for yourself nourishes your spirit as well as your body. As a busy mom, I've learned that when I don't take care of myself, I can't be fully present for my children and husband. When I sleep, make time for exercise, eat well, and do things I enjoy like writing or reading, I'm a much more pleasant person to be around! I also feel healthier and more in tune with my body. It's not selfish to put yourself first because, in doing so, you're actually better able to care for others. You're more grounded, you feel better, and you have a more optimistic outlook on life. When you put yourself on the back burner, you feel frazzled and your life becomes frenzied. This translates directly to your health and to your relationships with others.

One of my favorite quotes by Marianne Williamson in *A Course in Miracles* goes,

> *We are all meant to shine, as children do. We were*
> *born to make manifest the glory of God that is within us.*
> *It's not just in some of us; it's in everyone. And as we let*

our own light shine, we unconsciously give other people permission to do the same. As we are liberated from our own fear, our presence automatically liberates others.

So, don't feel guilty. Make yourself a priority. It serves everyone well.

---

* Anticancer Action *

Turn off your electronic devices and TV each night at least 30 minutes before you go to bed. Make sleep a priority.

Begin waking up 30 minutes earlier each morning to devote time to *yourself*. Exercise, read something inspiring, do devotions, write in your gratitude journal, or plan your to-do list. Bask in the quiet time of contemplation. You will automatically feel more grounded and ready to take on the day.

Chapter 10: Screenings for Cancer Prevention and Diagnosis

Throughout this book, we've discussed a myriad of ways to prevent cancer and other diseases. We know that diet and lifestyle play huge roles in deterring cancer formation. However, despite our best practices and intentions, cancer sometimes can still lurk in our bodies, especially if we have genetic predispositions. Therefore, it is of utmost importance to have cancer screenings performed at certain points in our lives, depending on our age and our gender.

One of the beauties of modern medicine is its capability for disease prevention. The face of cancer research is constantly changing. New drugs and therapies for cancer prevention and treatment are being researched and released on an ever-evolving basis. We also have diagnostic tools at our fingertips, most of which are covered by insurance. We need only make an appointment with our doctors, and screening tests can be ordered.

Based on our age and gender, a number of tests may be ordered to detect our susceptibility for various kinds of cancer. Cancer screening looks for cancer before a person has any symptoms. Screening tests can help find cancer at an early stage, before symptoms appear and/or before metastasis occurs. When abnormal tissue or cancer is found early, it may be easier to treat or cure. This is why early diagnosis is so critical to our health and longevity.

Different types of screening mechanisms exist. Some screenings are as simple as physical exams and patient history checklist. Others may be through blood draws or genetic testing. And other screenings are imaging procedures like MRIs or sonograms.

Most screening tests are benign, but as we will see, others have risks associated with them. One must weigh the options of getting the test versus not knowing of a potential cancer risk. There are also possible false-positive test results and false-negative test results. Screenings are not perfect, however most can be life-saving for many individuals.

In this chapter, we'll look at some recommended cancer screening tests. We'll assess their benefits as well as their potential complications or risks. We'll also look at second cancers (cancers that develop after a person has already had a primary cancer diagnosis) and how those may be precipitated or prevented.

Part One: Primary Cancers

1) Colorectal Cancer

Statistics: Colorectal cancer is the third most commonly diagnosed cancer in both men and women. It is also the second leading cause of cancer death in the United States.

Risk Factors: Causes and risk factors of this cancer vary. Some people may be genetically predisposed to developing colorectal cancer. Other risk factors include being over 50, overweight, diabetic, and sedentary. African-Americans are at a slightly higher risk. Those with inflammatory bowel conditions like Crohn's or colitis have a greater risk. Eating a low-fiber diet, smoking, and excessive alcohol consumption are also risk factors.

Symptoms: Symptoms of colorectal cancer include a change in bowel habits like more frequent diarrhea or constipation, rectal bleeding, black or tarry stools, abdominal pain or cramping, weakness and fatigue, and unexplained weight loss. Often, these symptoms may not present until cancer is already present. Early stages of cancer and benign polyps typically are asymptomatic.

Screenings:

* Sigmoidoscopy:

Regular screening is one of the most powerful weapons for preventing colorectal cancer. One option for screening is a sigmoidoscopy. If a person is age 50 or older and has no colon cancer risk factors other than age, which puts one at average risk, the doctor may recommend a flexible sigmoidoscopy exam every five years to screen for colon cancer.

A sigmoidoscopy examines the distal part of the colon only using a thin, flexible tube with a camera. The prep for this is easier than a colonoscopy and the patient needs not be sedated.

* Colonoscopy:

A colonoscopy is a more thorough evaluation and involves looking at the entire inner lining of a person's colon and rectum with the same type of scope. Doctors look for changes at the cellular level. If polyps are found, they can be removed during the colonoscopy and sent for biopsy. The doctor will also look for ulcers, tumors, and any source of bleeding.

Colonoscopies are recommended for those over 50 who are not at an increased risk for colorectal cancer. For those with an elevated risk, regular screening may begin in the 40s or even earlier, depending on doctor recommendations and whether or not the person is symptomatic. If nothing abnormal is found during colonoscopy, the test need not be repeated for 5-10 years. Again, your doctor will make recommendations for that based on risk factors and any symptoms. For anyone with polyps or abnormal findings, the test may be repeated sooner.

If polyps are found during a colonoscopy, they can be immediately removed. The great news is, most polyps take 10-15 years to become cancerous. So, early diagnosis and removal can prevent cancer from forming. It's estimated that 60% of colorectal cancer deaths can be prevented.

What are the risks of having a colonoscopy? Colonoscopy is generally a safe procedure, and because it's prescribed infrequently (every 5-10 years), the benefits typically outweigh any risks. However, colonoscopies can result in tears to the colon, heavy bleeding, inflammation, or infection. The test also requires sedation, so there's a possibility for an adverse reaction to medication. In order to prepare for a colonoscopy, one must also drink a laxative or take pills which helps to evacuate the bowel. This is difficult for some people, especially for those with limited movement or disability. Those with diabetes also may need to adjust exogenous insulin and/or may experience blood sugar imbalances. Those with low blood pressure may experience lightheadedness from the preparation. There is also some radiation involved as colonoscopies are done under fluoroscopy or x-ray.

Ultimately, colonoscopies can directly prevent cancer by the removal of polyps. Because they are recommended so infrequently for most people, the pros are greater than any cons.

2) Breast Cancer

Statistics: About one in eight U.S. women (about 12%) will develop invasive breast cancer over the course of her lifetime. Breast cancer is the second leading cause of cancer death in women following lung cancer. Only heart disease trumps cancer in death rates for women. Invasive breast cancer can be prevented, however, if caught early enough. If breast cancer is found only in breast tissue, the five-year survival rate after treatment is 99%. If cancer has spread to lymph nodes, the five-year survival rate is 85%. If the cancer has spread throughout the body, the five-year survival rate is 26%. The good news is, only 5% of women have metastatic cancer when they are first diagnosed.

Risk Factors: Risk factors for breast cancer include being overweight or sedentary; smoking; eating an unhealthy diet; drinking alcohol; using hormone replacement therapy after menopause; being on higher dose birth control pills; having a personal history of radiation to the chest or face; and having exposures to harmful chemicals in water, food, and the environment. Emerging science has linked low vitamin D levels with potential breast cancer risk. Also, light exposure at night, as with those who work night shifts, is a risk factor as natural circadian rhythms are disturbed.

However, some risk factors are out of one's control such as just being a woman, one's age, one's race, and genetic factors or family history. Having no children or having children after age 30 increases a woman's risk. Breastfeeding a child especially for more than a year can lower risk. Early menstruation, before age 12, is also a risk factor as is late menopause, over age 55. As we shall see, having dense breasts increases a woman's risk of developing breast cancer.

Symptoms: For most women with breast cancer, no symptoms are present which is why breast cancer is so scary and can be so invasive. Some women may feel a "lump" during a self-breast exam or at a physician's appointment. Others may experience pain in the breast or nipple, swelling in part of the breast, skin irritation or dimpling, nipple retraction, or nipple discharge (other than milk). If breast cancer has spread to lymph nodes under the arms or around the collar bone, they may become swollen or tender. Any abnormal symptoms should always be reported to a doctor.

Since 2007, death rates from breast cancer in women over 50 have declined. This is believed to be the result of finding breast cancer earlier through screening and increased awareness, as well as better treatments. Breast cancer rates in younger women have held steady, and this is probably due to genetic predispositions and/or lack of screening in younger women.

There are various screening methods for breast cancer. Mammograms have been the standard form of evaluation for decades, but there are also some different and/or newer screenings available which may or may not be covered by insurance.

Screenings:

* Mammograms:

Typically, women over age 40 are recommended for annual mammograms. Those with a family history of breast cancer may be screened earlier. A mammogram is a low-dose x-ray that allows specialists to look for changes in breast tissue. The x-rays are taken from at least two different angles to ensure that all breast tissue is seen. The machine has two plates that compress or flatten the breast to spread the tissue apart. These are standard mammograms. There are also 3D mammograms. The 3D mammogram compresses the breast once and takes numerous pictures, but it also has a higher level of radiation exposure.

Mammograms look for calcifications and masses. If an area of suspicion is found, doctors may recommend that a woman have a biopsy in which a needle is inserted into the area and cellular tissue withdrawn. The tissue would then be assessed for any cancer growth.

Mammogram screenings for breast cancer have been shown to reduce mortality from the disease among women ages 40 to 74, especially those age 50 or older. Overall, mammograms have an 84% sensitivity, meaning that mammography correctly identifies about 84% of women who truly have breast cancer.

Sensitivity is also better in older women and in those with fattier breast tissue. The opposite of fatty breast tissue is dense breast tissue. Having dense breasts means that a women has more breast and connective tissue than fat. Unfortunately, denser breast tissue makes reading a mammogram more difficult, and cancer can sometimes be left undetected in denser tissue. Often, younger women may have denser breasts. Some women also have a genetic predisposition toward denser breasts. Breast density may also be related to weight, age, number of pregnancies, or postmenopausal hormone use. Density is sometimes seen as a risk factor for cancer. According to the Susan G. Komen foundation, women with very dense breasts are four to five times more likely to develop breast cancer than women with low breast density. The exact reason for this is still unknown.

Women with denser breasts may need yearly mammograms and/or other screenings to help evaluate the tissue and to better determine if any cancerous tissue exists. These women should also be sure to perform breast self-examinations regularly.

As far as any risk factors go, mammograms are generally regarded as safe and can be life-saving for millions of women. However, there are some risk factors to consider. The Mayo Clinic lists the following risks and limitations: exposure to low-dose radiation (which is something to consider when getting annual mammograms); false-negative and false-positive results (mammograms may miss detecting some cancers especially in dense tissue, or women may go on to have multiple mammograms or a biopsy only to find that no cancer is present); and inability to accurately interpret mammograms especially in younger women.

Based on personal and family history, a woman over 40 might decide to have annual mammograms or to do them less frequently. Currently, guidelines vary across different organizations. The National Comprehensive Cancer Network recommends yearly mammograms for women beginning at age 40. However, the American Cancer Society recommends consultation with a doctor from ages 40-45 with yearly mammograms beginning at age 45. The U.S. Preventative Services Task Force recommends informed decision-making with a doctor about mammograms from ages 40-49 and mammograms every two years after age 50. Waiting until a later age for mammograms is considered because there are many false-positive results in younger women largely because they tend to have denser breasts. And overall, younger women have a lower risk of developing breast cancer than older women. Again, one's decision to have or not have a mammogram should be discussed with a doctor. All risk factors should be considered and part of the decision.

* **Breast MRI:**

A woman with a strong family history of breast cancer and/or who carries the BRCA1 or BRCA2 gene may be prescribed a breast magnetic resonance imaging (MRI) along with a mammogram. Screening with mammography plus breast MRI is not recommended for women at average risk of breast cancer. A breast MRI may also often be used for women with an existing cancer diagnosis to determine staging of the cancer.

Breast MRI uses magnetic fields to create an image of the breast. It is more invasive than mammography because a contrast agent is given through an IV before the procedure. The solution will help any potentially cancerous breast tissue show up more clearly.

The breast MRI does NOT use x-rays, so there is no radiation exposure risk. However, there is a greater risk for false-positive results. There may also be risk for false-negatives as the MRI does not pick up areas of calcification which can be a sign of cancer.

Typically, breast MRIs are not covered by insurance in women with average risk. They are also much more expensive than mammograms. This is why only a subset of women who have greater risk or already have a breast cancer diagnosis are approved for MRI.

* **Breast Ultrasound:**

A breast ultrasound (or sonogram) uses sound waves to produce pictures of the internal structures of the breast. It is noninvasive and does not use ionizing radiation. Ultrasound gel is placed directly onto the skin, and a transducer or probe is used to glide over the gel and breast tissue. High-frequency sound waves are transmitted from the probe through the gel into the body. This creates images, and blood circulation through vessels can also be seen.

Breast ultrasounds are primarily used to help diagnose breast lumps or other abnormalities a doctor may have found during a physical exam. The ultrasound can help determine if an area of concern is a fluid-filled cyst or a solid tumor.

Typically, a mammography would be completed first. If an area of suspicion is identified, a physician may order an ultrasound. (An MRI and ultrasound would not usually both be completed, but one or the other.)

Ultrasound may also be offered for women who are at higher risk for breast cancer. If a woman is pregnant and needs evaluation, an ultrasound would be used in lieu of mammography. Also, if a woman has very dense breasts, ultrasound may be ordered to more clearly see what is glandular and what is connective tissue. Also, if a woman has breast implants, an ultrasound may get a better view of lumps and cysts than a mammogram. Lastly, ultrasound is used to perform a guided biopsy.

The downside to breast ultrasound is that it may miss small lumps or solid tumors that are seen on mammography. Also, in women with very large breasts or in obese women, an ultrasound may miss visualization of tumors or calcification. Breast ultrasound alone is not a good technique for detection of breast cancer, but in conjunction with mammography, it can be quite useful.

* **Breast Thermography:**

Breast thermography is a 15-minute non-invasive test of physiology. It is painless and without any exposure to radiation. Breast thermography uses Digital Infrared Imaging (DII). This involves utilizing ultra-sensitive medical infrared cameras and sophisticated computers to detect, analyze, and produce high-resolution images of temperature variations. DII is based on the principle that metabolic activity and vascular circulation in both pre-cancerous tissue and the area surrounding a developing breast cancer is almost always higher than in normal breast tissue. So "hot spots" or areas that appear red on thermography potentially contain pre-cancerous or cancerous tissue.

Because the test is very sensitive, it can detect very early changes or signs of breast cancer. Researchers recommend having a baseline breast thermography as early as age 25. Thermography may be repeated yearly to detect minute changes in vasculature and tissue. Thermography can also see areas of angiogenesis (new blood vessel formation to tumor cells). A benefit of thermography is that areas of dense breast tissue do not interfere with the results. Canadian researchers found that thermography found 83% of breast cancer cells. This rivals those found on mammography.

Other benefits of thermography is that it exudes no radiation, and it is non-invasive. It also involves no compression of the breast. Although insurance does not currently cover thermography, it is relatively low-cost. One thermography session costs about $200 and takes 15-30 minutes.

The American Cancer Society and the FDA do not recommend thermography alone at this time but note that it can supplement mammograms. As with other forms of screening, thermography is not 100% accurate. It may still miss cancerous areas.

* Breast Cancer Gene (BRCA) Testing:

If a woman has a strong family history of breast cancer and/or a family member who has tested positive for a BRCA gene mutation, she may be advised to have this blood test completed. A woman's risk of both breast and ovarian cancer are increased if she tests positive for a BRCA1 or BRCA2 mutation. Only about 5-10% of breast and ovarian cancers are linked to the BRCA1 or BRCA2 gene changes, and only about two or three out of every thousand adult women have a BRCA gene change. Thus, this test is not commonly ordered. Only those with high risk factors would be tested. Most insurance companies will cover the cost of genetic testing if a person meets the conditions for testing.

Those who may be more likely to have a BRCA gene mutation include women (and immediate family members) diagnosed with breast cancer before age 50; those who've had breast cancer in both breasts; those who've had both breast and ovarian cancer; those with one or more *male* family members who've had breast cancer; and people who are Ashkenazi

Jews. Having one or several of these risk factors does not necessarily mean a person carries the mutated gene. Also, even if one does carry the gene mutation, this is not necessarily a cancer sentence.

If a woman tests positive for a BRCA gene change, she has about a 41-90% chance of getting breast cancer at some time in her life and about an 8-62% chance of getting ovarian cancer at some point. Knowing these odds can help one make informed decisions about prevention and health care.

Those with a BRCA gene mutation should still be able to get health insurance and it should not interfere with one's chance for employment. In the United States, there is a law called the Genetic Information Nondiscrimination Act of 2008 (GINA) which protects those with DNA mutations or differences. However, this law does not protect against discrimination in life insurance, disability insurance, or long-term care insurance.

Women with the BRCA mutation sometimes opt for prophylactic mastectomies (removal of one or both breasts). This has been found to reduce the risk of breast cancer in high-risk women by about 90%. Others may opt for prophylactic salpingo-oophorectomy, or removal of both ovaries and fallopian tubes. This can reduce breast cancer risk by as much as 50% when it is done before menopause, because it takes away the body's main source of the hormone estrogen. It also obviously reduces the risk of ovarian cancer. For those with a BRCA1 abnormality, the recommended timing of removing both ovaries and fallopian tubes is between ages 35 and 40. For those with a BRCA2 abnormality, removing ovaries and fallopian tubes can be considered between ages 40 and 45. There are also some hormonal therapies that may be effective in warding off cancer. Among them are Tamoxifen, Evista, Aromasin, and Arimidex. Each has its own role in preventing hormone-receptor positive cancers. They are not without risks or side effects, so conversation with one's doctor is of utmost importance in determining course of action.

It goes without saying that women who test positive for BRCA1 or BRCA2 mutations should seek early and frequent screening for breast cancer. For those women, these are life-saving measures.

* Breast Self-Exam:

Every adult woman should be performing monthly breast self-exams. According to Johns Hopkins Medical Center, 40% of diagnosed breast cancers are found by women who feel a lump. Mammograms are effective in determining many cancer cases before they become lumps. But when a woman is familiar with the natural contours of her breast and recognizes changes, she can immediately alert a healthcare professional.

Several days after a woman's monthly cycle ends, her breasts are likely to be fuller and more tender. This is a good time for a self-check. If a woman is no longer having a period, she can just choose a day each month, like the first of the month, to perform the exam.

Doctors recommend doing the exam in the shower where the fingers can easily move over wet skin. Using the pads of your fingers, move around the entire breast in a circular pattern moving from the outside to the center, checking the entire breast and armpit area for hardened areas, lumps, or thickening. Standing in front of the mirror is another good option since a woman can look for dimpling, swelling, etc. Sometimes doctors also recommend lying down to perform the check since the breast tissue spreads out easily.

Breast self-exams are easy, relatively quick, and free. There really is no excuse not to do a monthly check. Of course, these should not replace other forms of screening like mammography, but self-exams can be useful in between mammography screenings.

3) Ovarian Cancer

Statistics: In the United States, ovarian cancer strikes about 22,000 women each year. It ranks fifth in cancer deaths among women. A woman's risk for ovarian cancer is about 1 in 75 throughout the course of her lifetime.

Risk Factors: As a woman ages, her chances of developing ovarian cancer increase. Half of all ovarian cancers are found in women 63 years of age or older. Age is an unavoidable risk factor as are genetic conditions. As we discussed in regard to breast cancer, having BRCA gene mutations may predispose women to developing ovarian cancer as well. Other risk factors include obesity, use of fertility drugs, postmenopausal hormone therapy, personal history of breast cancer before age 40, and a family history of the disease. Women who have never given birth or who had their first baby after the age of 35 are at increased risk. Breastfeeding appears to *decrease* the risk of ovarian cancer, as does use of oral contraceptives. Women who've had a tubal ligation (tubes tied) may have a reduced chance of developing ovarian cancer by up to two-thirds. Having a hysterectomy also seems to reduce the risk for ovarian cancer by up to one-third.

Symptoms: Unfortunately, ovarian cancer is often a silent killer. Many women do not have symptoms until the cancer has progressed and spread beyond the ovaries. However, there are some telltale signs of this cancer. The most common symptoms include bloating, pelvic or abdominal pain, trouble eating or feeling full quickly, and urinary urgency and frequency. Other symptoms include fatigue, nausea, back pain, pain during sex, constipation, menstrual changes, and abdominal swelling with weight loss. The problem with many of these symptoms is that they could also be attributed to other conditions or to benign illnesses. If a woman experiences persistent and recurring changes, she should seek immediate medical advice. Only about 20% of ovarian cancers are found in the early stages. Early detection is critical and probably life-saving.

Screenings:

* CA-125 Blood Test:

CA-125 (cancer antigen 125) is a protein in the blood. Initially, this test was used as a tumor marker. Levels are increased with an ovarian cancer diagnosis. If an elevated CA-125 decreases with cancer treatment, this can indicate the treatment is working.

More recently, CA-125 may also be used to detect the early stages of ovarian cancer in a woman at higher risk. The problem with this screening, however, is that other conditions can also elevate CA-125, giving false-positive results. Some of the conditions which could throw off the CA-125 test are endometriosis, menstruation, liver disease, pregnancy, uterine fibroids, and pelvic inflammatory disease. Some other cancers might also elevate CA-125 such as those of the uterus or fallopian tube. Because of its possible unreliability, the CA-125 blood test is not deemed accurate enough to be used for all women. If a woman has a strong family history of ovarian cancer and/or carries a BRCA gene mutation, she may be a good candidate for this screening.

* Transvaginal Ultrasound:

Transvaginal ultrasound (TVUS) is a test that uses sound waves to look at the uterus, fallopian tubes, and ovaries by putting an ultrasound wand into the vagina. It can help detect masses in the ovaries or fluid-filled cysts.

In a study that followed more than 14,000 women over 12 years, researchers performed annual TVUS on the women. The study included women who were either age 30 or older with a family history of ovarian cancer, or age 50 or older. Researchers found that annual transvaginal ultrasound screening permitted early detection of most ovarian cancers and improved five-year survival from about 50% to 88% in screened patients.

There is little risk to having a TVUS. No radiation is used. This is an internal exam, however, so a woman would need to disrobe and expect to have the ultrasound probe inserted into her vagina two to three inches. This should not cause any discomfort. Often a woman is advised to drink at least 32 ounces of fluid beforehand. Having a full bladder allows the intestines to be lifted to get a better picture of the ovaries. It may be somewhat uncomfortable for a woman to hold her urine throughout the procedure.

4) Cervical Cancer

Statistics: Cervical cancer death rates have dropped by 50% over the last 40 years. This is largely attributed to increased screenings. Each year, about 12,000 women are diagnosed with cervical cancer. Cervical pre-cancers are diagnosed far more often than invasive cervical cancer. Pre-cancers are sometimes referred to as dysplasia. Each year, up to a million women are diagnosed with dysplasia. Most dysplasia can be treated and cervical cancer prevented.

Risk Factors: The biggest risk factor for cervical cancer is exposure to the human papilloma virus (HPV). HPV is the most common sexually transmitted disease. HPV is so common that nearly all sexually active people get it at some point in their lives. Most often, HPV will go away on its own. However, certain strains of the virus cause issues like genital warts or cervical cancer. Besides having HPV, some other risk factors for cervical cancer are smoking, oral contraceptive use, herpes infection, family history, early pregnancy (before age 17) or more than three pregnancies, race/ethnicity (African Americans and Hispanics are at greater risk), and having a lowered immunity (caused by things like corticosteroid use, cancer treatment, organ transplantation, or the HIV virus).

Symptoms: In the early stages of the disease, cervical cancer does not likely cause any symptoms. If symptoms do present, a woman may experience vaginal bleeding, abnormal vaginal discharge, or pelvic pain, especially during intercourse. If the cancer is advanced and/or metastasized, a woman may experience weight loss, fatigue, back pain, leg swelling, leaking of urine through the vaginal opening, or even bone fractures.

Screenings:

* Pap Smear:

A Pap smear is performed during a routine gynecological exam. The doctor will gently scrape cells from the surface of the cervix. The tissue sample is then sent for testing to determine the presence of abnormal cells or dysplasia.

Typically, a women will have her first Pap smear between the ages of 18 and 21. This is usually an annual procedure (or once every three years) until the age of 30. After age 30, if a woman has had three consecutive normal Pap smears, her doctor may recommend repeating the test every five years, as long as no new sexual partners have been introduced. After the age of 65, a woman may no longer need to have the Pap smear test completed.

If a woman does have dysplasia, Pap smears may be repeated every six months. Depending on the degree of dysplasia, further testing may be done. The doctor may recommend a **colposcopy**. During this procedure, a doctor inserts a tool called a colposcope which looks like binoculars with a bright light mounted to it. It gives the physician a better view of the cervix and surrounding tissue. The doctor may also take a biopsy at that time to determine the invasiveness and severity of the dysplasia. If the cervical dysplasia remains after a colposcopy, the doctor may recommend having a **LEEP** (loop electrosurgical excision procedure). A fine wire with low-voltage electrical current can remove the abnormal tissue form the cervix. There are other methods of cervical tissue extraction as well, but this is the primary way and can be completed in the physician's office.

There are really no risks to having a Pap smear completed. False-negative results are possible, which is why routine testing for a period of time is recommended. Colposcopy with a biopsy has relatively few risks. However, because it is more invasive, there are risks for bleeding, infection, pelvic pain, or cramping. The LEEP, being even more invasive, can have further risks. Along with infection and bleeding, a woman may have scarring of cervical tissue, trouble getting pregnant, or even risk for premature birth or low birth weight as the woman's cervix may have been thinned or compromised from removal of tissue. Although the benefits of screening and removal of dysplastic tissue probably outweigh the risks, a woman should be aware of these possible outcomes.

Both the LEEP and cone biopsies (colposcopies) are 85-90% effective in treating moderate to severely abnormal cells of the cervix. The majority of patients who have abnormal Pap smears and then are treated with a LEEP or cone biopsy subsequently have normal Pap smears.

* HPV Testing:

The HPV test detects the presence of human papillomavirus, a virus that can lead to the development of genital warts, abnormal cervical cells, or cervical cancer. A doctor may recommend having this test completed if a woman has an abnormal Pap smear and/or is over the age of 30. Because HPV is so common, especially in younger women, it will likely be detected in that population. The good news is the virus can clear on its own in one to two years. However, if a woman deals with this after a period of time, closer attention must be paid.

The HPV test can be done simultaneously with the Pap test, even using the same cellular tissue samples. Like the Pap smear, the HPV test is just a gentle swab removal of surface cells. A Pap test plus an HPV test (called co-testing) is the preferred way to find early cervical cancer or precancerous cells in women over 30. Co-screening is beneficial because it means fewer tests, follow-up visits, and treatments may be needed. According to the American Cancer Society, it usually takes more than 10 years for cell changes to become cancer, so if a woman has a normal Pap and HPV test, her chance of developing cancer between exams is minimal.

For more information on HPV transmission as well as on vaccination for HPV, please refer back to Chapter 8.

5) Prostate Cancer

Statistics: The prostate is a small gland that sits below a man's bladder. The prostate gland may be susceptible to cancer because of its role in male reproduction and hormones. About one in seven men will be diagnosed with prostate cancer during their lifetime. Next to skin cancer, prostate cancer is the most commonly diagnosed cancer in men. This cancer is uncommon in men under 40. The average age of diagnosis is 66. Prostate cancer is the third leading cause of cancer death in American men, behind lung cancer and colorectal cancer. Prostate cancer can be a serious disease, but the good news is most men diagnosed with prostate cancer do not die from it.

Risk Factors: Prostate cancer risk increases with age. Certain ethnicities also appear to have a larger risk. African-American and Caribbean men of African descent are more likely to develop the disease as well as to die from it. Asian men have the lowest risk. Sometimes prostate cancer can run in families, although the majority of cases are in men with no family history. Some genetic factors may play into the development of this cancer. A family history of BRCA gene mutations and other genetic anomalies may increase a man's risk. Obesity, smoking, exposure to harmful chemicals, and diet may all play a role. Some studies have shown that diets high in calcium and dairy may also increase risk.

Symptoms: Prostate cancer may have no symptoms. However, some men experience bleeding or pain during urination, difficulty urinating or trouble starting and stopping flow, frequency, and loss of bladder control. If the cancer has metastasized, a man may experience pain in the spine; painful or bloody ejaculation; swelling in legs or pelvis; numbness in the hip, legs, or feet; or bone pain that doesn't go away or leads to fractures.

Screenings:

* Prostate Specific Antigen (PSA):

A man's PSA can be tested through blood work. PSA is a protein produced by both cancerous and noncancerous tissue in the prostate. Small amounts of PSA ordinarily circulate in men's blood. If a man's PSA is elevated, this may signify the presence of cancer. However, many other conditions, such as an enlarged or inflamed prostate, can also increase PSA levels. Therefore, determining what a high PSA score means can be complicated. An elevated PSA is not a diagnostic tool for cancer, but it can guide a doctor's focus for further testing.

* Digital Rectal Exam (DRE):

During a DRE, a doctor inserts a lubricated, gloved finger into the rectum to reach the prostate. By feeling or pressing on the prostate, the doctor may be able to judge whether it has abnormal lumps or hard areas. A DRE may be performed yearly as a part of a man's routine annual check-up. Like the PSA, a DRE is not a diagnostic tool, but an abnormal finding may lead a doctor to recommend having a biopsy. During this procedure, samples of tissue are removed for laboratory examination. A diagnosis of cancer is based on the biopsy results.

Professional organizations differ in their recommendations for PSA testing. Some do not have definitive guidelines. Organizations that do recommend PSA screening generally encourage the test in men between the ages of 40 and 70, and in men with an increased risk of prostate cancer. Men may only need to be tested every two years if the PSA is low (less than 2.5 ng/ml). In a higher PSA range, a man may be tested yearly.

The pros of PSA testing are that it can detect cancer early, making it easier to treat; it is a simple blood test; and by knowing a man's PSA number, it may prevent the spread of cancer and death. The cons of PSA testing are that some cancers are slow growing and never extend beyond the prostate gland, possibly manifesting as a low PSA count even in the presence of cancer. Another concern is that not all prostate cancers need treatment, but a physician may be more apt to treat the cancer if found. Surgery and treatment for prostate cancer can result in temporary or permanent incontinence and erectile dysfunction. Every man must weigh the pros and cons and discuss the potential benefits of PSA testing with his doctor.

6) Skin Cancer

Statistics: Skin cancer is the most common type of cancer in the United States. One in five Americans will develop some form of skin cancer during their lifetime. There are three main types of skin cancer: basal cell carcinoma, squamous cell carcinoma, and melanoma. Of the three, melanoma is the deadliest.

Typically, basal cell and squamous cell carcinomas can be removed with minor surgery and cured during the process. Dermatologists can perform these excisions. Rarely, these cancers might become more advanced, especially if left untreated, and may require radiation and even chemotherapy. However, this is unlikely.

Melanoma accounts for less than one percent of skin cancer cases, but the vast majority of skin cancer deaths. When melanoma is detected early, the five-year survival rate is about 98%. The survival rate falls to 62% when the disease reaches the lymph nodes, and 18% when the disease metastasizes to distant organs.

Risk Factors: Risk factors for skin cancer largely focus around sun exposure and a personal history of sunburns. One UK study found that about 86% of melanomas can be attributed to exposure to ultraviolet (UV) radiation from the sun. It's also estimated that about 90% of non-melanoma skin cancers are a direct result of sun exposure. Tanning in tanning beds is also a major risk factor. More than 419,000 cases of skin cancer in the U.S. each year are linked to indoor tanning. Other risk factors include having a fair complexion and/or blue or green eyes, a family history of skin cancer, many moles and/or abnormal moles, exposure to radiation for skin conditions, and a weakened immune system.

Symptoms: What are the symptoms of skin cancer? Non-melanoma skin cancers typically present as an unusual skin growth, bump, or sore that doesn't go away. It can be waxy and translucent or discolored or darkly pigmented. It can be rough and scaly or smooth. Sometimes a cancerous basal or squamous cell carcinoma may not look much different from the normal surrounding skin. Melanomas appear as new moles or spots that change in size, shape, or color. The ABCDE rule is a helpful reference for examining moles and areas of skin change to identify whether or not melanoma is present. "A" stands for asymmetry. The mole may be an uneven or imperfect shape. "B" is for border. A suspicious mole's border may be irregular or ragged. "C" is for color. The color may include different shades within the same mole. "D" is for diameter. The diameter of a melanoma is often more than 6 mm. And "E" is for evolving. This means the mole keeps changing in size, shape, and color. Sometimes these suspicious moles may also ooze, itch, cause pain or tenderness, or swell.

Screenings:

* Skin Exam:

Dermatologists often recommend yearly skin checks for their patients. A person should always be looking for any changes in their skin or areas of concern. Having a professional also examine the entire body can ensure skin cancers are found early.

During a skin exam, a patient would disrobe. The doctor will check any areas of concern and also look at the rest of a person's skin. Skin cancer can hide in strange places like between toes, on the bottom of feet, under the hair on the scalp, under fingernails, in and around ears, on the lips, and even on the genitalia. The doctor may also feel the lymph nodes around areas of concern or in the neck, underarm, and groin area. Enlarged lymph nodes can indicate the spread of melanoma.

* Excision and Biopsy:

There is a risk that doctors may "over-treat" a patient, removing more moles and suspicious areas than necessary. However, it's best to be proactive when it comes to skin cancer because skin cancers found and removed early are almost always curable.

Excision of the area often completely removes any cancerous or pre-cancerous cells. A doctor may choose to send the cells for biopsy. If the biopsy is positive for cancer, further excision or treatment may be needed. If melanoma is found, surrounding lymph nodes may also be biopsied, and imaging procedures like MRIs or CT scans may be performed to determine severity. Metastatic melanoma may require other treatments, too, such as chemotherapy, radiation, interferon, or immunotherapy.

7) Lung Cancer

Statistics: Lung cancer is the second most common form of cancer in both men and women, but it is the leading cause of death for both genders. About one in four cancer deaths are directly or indirectly related to lung cancer.

Lung cancer occurs mostly in people older than 65. Only 2% of lung cancer cases are in people under age 45.

Risk Factors: By far the greatest risk factor for lung cancer is smoking. It's estimated that 80% of lung cancer cases are directly related to smoking. The longer someone smokes and the more packs-per-day smoked correspondingly increases risk. Cigarettes are the greatest contributor due to their present and past popularity, however cigar and pipe smoking also increase one's risk for lung cancer. Secondhand smoke is also thought to cause more than 7,000 deaths from lung cancer each year.

The second largest contributor to lung cancer is exposure to radon. Radon is a colorless and odorless naturally occurring radioactive gas that results from the breakdown of uranium in soil and rocks. Radon can seep into one's home without the homeowner even knowing it. Breathing it in exposes ones lungs to small amounts of radiation which, over time, accumulates.

Another risk factor is exposure to asbestos. In recent years, government regulations have greatly reduced the use of asbestos in commercial and industrial products. But it's still present in many homes and other older buildings. This is why when one is doing major home renovation or demolition, a reliable asbestos abatement company should be utilized to prevent the asbestos from leaking into the air.

Other harmful chemicals like uranium, arsenic, vinyl chloride, nickel compounds, and coal products may also be hazardous to the lungs. This is especially true for industrial workers who deal with these materials. Air and water pollution are also risk factors. Some researchers estimate that about 5% of all deaths from lung cancer worldwide may be due to outdoor air pollution. Societies in which arsenic is present in the drinking water experience higher levels of lung cancer.

Other risk factors include previous radiation to the chest, such as for breast cancer or Hodgkin's disease. A family history of lung cancer may place one at higher risk. In Chapter 5, we discussed the dangers of taking beta-carotene if a person currently smoked or had a history of smoking. Researchers aren't sure why, but beta-carotene supplementation may harm smokers, further increasing their chances of developing lung cancer.

Symptoms: Often in the early stages, lung cancer has no symptoms. However, there are some hallmark symptoms to look for, especially if one has a susceptibility to developing lung cancer. A chronic cough that does not go away or worsens over time is a key indicator. Other symptoms include chest pain that is worse with coughing or deep breathing, coughing up blood, hoarseness, wheezing, loss of appetite, shortness of breath, fatigue, and recurrent bronchitis or pneumonia. If the cancer has spread, lymph nodes may be affected and enlarged. With metastatic cancer, a person may experience bone pain, jaundice, or neurological changes.

Screenings:

There is not a standard screening process for lung cancer. However, a doctor may advise some testing based on a patient's history.

* Low-dose helical or spiral computed tomography (CT) scan:

This CT scan creates a three-dimensional picture of the inside of the body. A computer then combines these images into a detailed, cross-sectional view that shows any abnormalities or tumors in the lungs. The U.S. Preventative Services Task Force recommends this scan yearly for those with a history of heavy smoking and who currently smoke or have quit in the last 15 years. Of that population, it's recommended for those 55-80 years old.

The National Lung Screening Trial (NLST) was a large clinical trial that looked at using low-dose CT scan of the chest to screen for lung cancer. It compared these CT scans with standard chest x-rays. People in the study got either three low-dose CT scans or three chest x-rays, each a year apart, to look for abnormal areas in the lungs that might be cancer. After several years, the study found that people who got CT scans had a 20% lower chance of dying from lung cancer than those who got chest x-rays. They were also 7% less likely to die overall (from any cause) than those who got chest x-rays. The CT scans are very detailed and can show early-stage lung cancers that may be too small to be detected by a traditional x-ray.

Compared to a conventional CT, the low-dose CT scan for lung cancer uses approximately five times less radiation. It is also a quick exam, lasting less than a minute.

The risks of having a low-dose CT scan are that doctors may find areas of concern that suggest lung cancer when no cancer is actually present. This may lead to unnecessary treatments and/or surgeries. False-positive results are not uncommon. Over-diagnosis is also possible. This occurs when small cancers are found that may not have caused problems or metastasized, but were treated anyway. This can affect the quality of life for individuals. Another risk is that even though these CT scans are low-dose, with yearly exposure, cancers can form as a result of radiation.

8) Liver Cancer

Statistics: Since 1980, the incidence of liver cancer has tripled. The liver, our largest internal organ, is being threatened by the increase in unhealthy lifestyles across the world. Alcoholism and Hepatitis B and C are root causes of cirrhosis as is fatty-liver disease which is often caused by an unhealthy diet, obesity, and diabetes. Cirrhosis increases one's odds of developing liver cancer. Liver cancer is the 10th most common cancer, and men are three times more likely to get the disease than women.

Risk Factors: As mentioned, there are some preventable risk factors. Eating a healthy diet and avoiding or limiting processed foods, sugars, and alcohol can create a better environment for the liver to thrive. This helps reduce the risk factors of cirrhosis and fatty-liver disease. Those infected with Hepatitis B and C, as mentioned, are at higher risk. There is a vaccination for Hepatitis B, and Hepatitis C can be prevented by practicing safe sex and avoiding contact with blood of infected individuals. Being obese and diabetic are also risk factors for liver cancer largely due to the association with fatty-liver disease. Long-term exposure to aflatoxins is a risk factor. Aflatoxins are cancer-causing substances are made by a fungus that contaminates peanuts, wheat, soybeans, ground nuts, corn, and rice. This is more common in tropical climates as aflatoxins grow in moist, warm environments. Some chemicals also increase the risk of liver cancer. Arsenic (in some drinking water) and vinyl chloride (in some plastics) are known liver toxins. Tobacco use is also associated with increased prevalence of liver cancer. Some risk factors like gender and race cannot be avoided. Men are at greater risk for developing liver cancer as are people of Asian descent and Pacific Islanders.

Symptoms: Symptoms of liver cancer often do not present for some time, thus the disease is sometimes called a "silent killer." Early stages of the disease may be asymptomatic. When symptoms appear, they may be vague and/or confused with other ailments. These symptoms include weight loss, loss of appetite, feeling full after a small meal, nausea and vomiting, enlarged spleen, enlarged liver, abdominal pain, pain in the right shoulder blade, itching, yellowish skin and eyes, and abnormal bruising and bleeding. Hormonal symptoms that can be caused by liver tumors include increasingly high cholesterol, high blood calcium, low blood sugar levels, gynecomastia (breast enlargement in men), and high red blood cells.

Screenings:

* Alph-fetoprotein (AFP) Blood Test:

Because liver cancer is so difficult to recognize in its early stages, doctors may recommend a blood test for at-risk patients. AFP is a protein made by the liver and yolk sac of the developing fetus and normally found in fetal blood. In healthy, non-pregnant adults, AFP blood levels are extremely low. An increased reading is a signal that something is wrong. Two-thirds of liver cancers produce AFP. If a person is at high risk, an AFP blood test may be ordered every six months.

The downfall of AFP testing is that other conditions can cause an elevation. As mentioned, pregnancy increases AFP as does cirrhosis of the liver. Other cancers may also raise the level of AFP. These cancers include testicular, ovarian, stomach, and pancreatic. If a person is diagnosed with liver cancer, AFP may be frequently tested to check the effectiveness of treatment and whether or not the levels drop in response to this treatment.

* Liver Ultrasound:

In addition to AFP testing, doctors recommend that people at high risk of liver cancer also have an ultrasound examination every six to twelve months. The ultrasound can help detect the presence of tumors on the liver. Elevated AFP with no liver lesion on the ultrasound means the patient probably has inflammation of the liver, not cancer. These patients should still be monitored closely. Interestingly and important to note, a patient may show a tumor on ultrasound, but not have an elevated AFP. So, ultrasounds are equally as important with or without AFP testing in high-risk patients.

Part Two: Second Cancers

A **secondary cancer** is a cancer which presents after a primary cancer diagnosis. A primary cancer is where a cancer starts. Sometimes cancer cells can break away from the primary cancer and settle and grow in another part of the body. This new cancer growth is called secondary cancer. The cells are the same as the first. For example, if a woman has breast cancer and later develops bone cancer, biopsies may show that the bone cancer is, in fact, just metastasis of the breast cancer. In other words, secondary cancer is a metastasis and/or a reoccurrence of the original cancer. Secondary cancer may occur simultaneously with the first cancer diagnosis, or it may present years later. Prevention of secondary cancer is to effectively treat the primary cancer and to hopefully catch it in its early stages before it spreads. This is precisely why screening is of utmost importance as is reporting to one's doctor any abnormal physical symptoms and illnesses.

Second cancers, on the other hand, are a brand new type of cancer, different from a person's first malignancy. (Sometimes in literature "second" and "secondary" cancers are used interchangeably, so it's important to pay attention to the context in which they're used.) If someone has had a primary cancer diagnosis, this does NOT mean they will go on to develop another cancer. After treatment, most individuals remain healthy and continue in remission from the first cancer. However, current research shows that cancer survivors, in general, have an increased chance of developing cancer compared to people of the same age and gender who have not had cancer. This means that it is even more important for cancer survivors to be aware of the risk factors for second cancers and maintain good follow-up health care.

Risk Factors for Second Cancers

* Cancer Treatments:

Often, second cancers may be a result of treatment from a primary cancer. These cancers can occur months, years, or even decades after treatment. Some treatments increase the risk of developing a second cancer, such as some chemotherapy drugs, radiation therapy for certain cancers, and treatment with both radiation therapy and chemotherapy together.

Although **chemotherapy and radiation** can be life-saving measures for those afflicted with cancer, they are also toxic poisons by nature and are carcinogenic in and of themselves. Chemotherapy destroys cancer cells, but it also affects normal cells. Some chemotherapy drugs seem to cause this more than others. For example, the drug Etoposide is associated with an increased risk of acute leukemia compared to other chemotherapy drugs. (Some other chemo drugs associated with a higher risk of second cancer include Procarbazine, Mechlorethamine, Chlorambucil, BCNU, Nitrogen mustard, Cyclophosphamide, Ifosfamide,

Epipodophyllotoxins, and Anthracyclines.) As far as radiation therapy goes, the higher dose given, the more likely to develop problems down the road. For survivors of childhood cancer, radiation therapy is the most important risk factor for second cancers. Also, the combined effects of chemo and radiation further increase the risk of developing a second cancer.

As an aside, chemotherapy and radiation are also known triggers for **Myelodysplastic Syndrome (MDS)**. Although not technically a cancer, MDS is considered a "preleukemia." It is a bone marrow disorder in which the bone marrow does not produce enough healthy blood cells. Instead, defective cells outnumber normal ones. This can result in anemia, bleeding, bruising, or severe infection. Well-known television anchor Robin Roberts, from *Good Morning America*, was diagnosed with this following chemo and radiation treatment. Roberts underwent a bone marrow transplant as well as further chemotherapy to treat the condition.

Incidentally, besides cancer, chemotherapy and radiation are also associated with other conditions or illnesses. These include heart disease, congestive heart failure, heart arrhythmias, high blood pressure, lung damage, early menopause in women, andropause in men, osteoporosis, infertility, thyroid issues, hearing loss, stroke, nervous system complications, and dental and vision impairments.

Having a **bone marrow transplant** as part of treatment also increases the odds for getting a second cancer. In addition to chemo and radiation that may have accompanied the transplant, the increased risk for second cancers may also be due to a compromised immune system and/or genetic abnormalities.

* Other Risk Factors:

Other risk factors for developing a second cancer exist. The age of treatment makes a big difference. Children and young adults have a higher risk of second cancers related to treatment with radiation or chemotherapy than older adults have. As we age, the risk of cancer increases for the general population but potentially even more so for cancer survivors.

A family history of cancer(s) increases one's odds of developing other cancers. Lifestyle is also a factor. Smoking, excessive sun exposure, a poor diet, obesity, lack of exercise, or excessive drinking after a primary cancer diagnosis can increase the chances of a second cancer outbreak.

Primary Cancers Prone to Second Cancer Development

A person can experience *any* cancer as a second cancer, and *any* primary cancer may make one more susceptible to getting a second. However, some cancers are more likely after the diagnosis and treatment of certain primary cancers.

Sometimes a second cancer can be relatively benign such as **skin cancer**. Squamous cell or basal cell carcinomas are common especially in those who've had childhood cancer. This may be due to radiation therapy. However, other second cancers are potentially deadly and/or just as aggressive as the first cancer.

* Hodgkin's disease:

Hodgkin's disease is one such primary cancer that is more likely to lead to a second cancer diagnosis. One study found the specific risk of dying from a second cancer after Hodgkin's disease was increased six times compared to the normal population. In patients treated when they were younger than 21 years of age, the risk was even greater with a 14-fold increase in death from a second cancer. The risk of second cancers was the greatest in those patients who required the most treatment. The most common cancers after Hodgkin's disease are **breast, thyroid, bone, colorectal, lung, stomach, leukemia, and lymphoma.**

* Breast Cancer:

After a primary diagnosis of breast cancer, women may be more susceptible to developing another breast cancer, especially in the other breast. Other, less prevalent cancers which may follow are **esophageal, stomach, salivary gland, colon, uterine, ovarian, thyroid, melanoma, and leukemia.**

* Non-Hodgkin's lymphoma (NHL):

NHL is another cancer with a higher than average second cancer rate. This increased risk continues for up to 20 years after treatment. The most common secondary cancers include **cancer of the lung, brain, kidney, or bladder; melanoma; leukemia; or Hodgkin's disease.**

* Acute Lymphoblastic Leukemia (ALL):

ALL is often a disease of childhood. In children, 80% with ALL are cured by treatments. But because of the radiation therapy, survivors of this cancer are more susceptible to a second cancer. In an evaluation of over 800 children who had survived ALL, those treated with radiation appeared to have a 20-fold increase compared to the general population. Some of those studied had a relapse of the ALL, while others developed a second cancer. These second cancers included **Acute Myeloid Leukemia (AML), lymphoma, basal cell carcinoma, other carcinomas, sarcoma, meningioma, and other brain tumors**.

* Testicular Cancer:

The chemotherapy that surrounds testicular cancer treatment may also lead to a second cancer diagnosis later. Patients may be at risk for **leukemia** after such treatment. Men diagnosed with testicular cancer are also at risk for developing **contra-lateral testicular cancer** (in the other testes).

Symptoms of Second Cancers

Because second cancers vary in type and degree of severity, symptoms will be different. However, anyone who has experienced a primary cancer diagnosis should always be on the lookout for any changes in his or her health.

Signs that cancer may be lurking in one's body include excessive fatigue, easy bruising or bleeding, paleness, bone pain, changes in moles, lumps, trouble swallowing, ongoing stomach pain, changes in bowel or bladder habits, blood in stools or urine, ongoing cough or hoarseness, shortness of breath, bloody sputum, mouth sores that don't heal, ongoing headaches, vision changes, and early morning vomiting.

Having any of the above symptoms does not necessarily mean that a person has cancer. However, if a person has more than one and/or the symptoms are persistent, a doctor should be notified.

Preventing Second Cancers

Knowing the symptoms of cancer is half the battle. If you've had a primary cancer, you'll need to be vigilant and aware of any changes in your health for the remainder of your life.

* Continued Cancer Screenings:

First and foremost, routine cancer checks are critical. Colonoscopies, mammograms, gynecological exams, digital rectal exams, and any doctor recommended blood work is essential in the prevention of second cancers.

* Choosing the Least Invasive Treatment:

Of course, if you've received a primary cancer diagnosis, you'll discuss with your doctor your treatment options and determine which action path is best. The *UNM Comprehensive Cancer Center* states, "The importance of defining risk groups is that less treatment can be given to those who have a low risk of recurrence of cancer with standard treatments and more treatment can be given to those at high risk. Lowering the dose of treatment for low risk groups is probably the most important way to prevent secondary cancers since these cancers occur more often in intensively treated patients." In other words, if your primary cancer was invasive and/or likely to reoccur or metastasize, treatment may be more aggressive. However, if the primary cancer was caught early and/or less likely to reoccur or spread, less treatment is preferred so as to avoid the harmful effects of chemo and radiation.

* Adjunct Therapies:

In conjunction with primary cancer treatments like chemo and/or radiation and/or surgery, other lifestyle additions may help with the success of treatment. There is some literature suggesting that **hyperbaric oxygen chambers** can help decrease the inflammatory process of radiation. It can boost the efficacy of chemotherapy as well. Also, cancer cells hate oxygen. By hyper-saturating cells with oxygen, cancerous cells can die off faster while healthy cells receive the nourishment they need.

Another lifestyle trend to try is following a **ketogenic diet**. We looked more extensively at this diet in Chapter 7. Ketogenic diets may be helpful in reducing the reoccurrence of cancer because they force the body to rely on ketones instead of sugar for energy. Remember that sugar is cancer's best friend. When the body is "starved" of simple sugars and carbohydrates, it turns to burning fat for fuel. Cancer cells cannot thrive well in this environment.

High-dose vitamin C therapy may slow or stop the growth of tumors. Studies have shown that vitamin C can prevent the onset or spread of prostate, pancreatic, liver, and colon cancers. IV vitamin C may also improve the quality of life for cancer patients. In a study published in *Free Radical Biology & Medicine,* vitamin C chelation therapy was found to be highly pro-oxidant after just one hour of treatment. This treatment provided beneficial long-term antioxidant effects in normal tissues and offered protection against carcinogenic insult. Vitamin C was responsible for destroying cancer cells.

Some other supplements to consider are **Frankincense essential oil, Holy Basil, and proteolytic enzyme therapy**. We'll not get into the inner workings of these therapies as they do require some research and consultation with a doctor. However, they are therapies to consider when taking a naturopathic approach to cancer healing and treatment. Proteolytic enzymes are thought to create an anti-inflammatory environment in the body. Holy Basil helps protect the body from radiation poisoning and heals damage from radiation treatment, and it increases the antioxidant glutathione. Frankincense is thought to have cancer-killing effects by influencing the genes to promote healing.

* Lifestyle Practices:

Other preventative tactics are similar to the prevention of primary cancers. Quitting smoking, drinking in moderation, protecting skin from overexposure to sun, following a healthy diet (as described in Chapter 2), taking appropriate supplements (as described in Chapter 4), losing weight when necessary, and exercising are some of the many ways to help prevent a second cancer. And never underestimate the power of prayer, friendships, gratitude, and laughter.

Final Thoughts on Cancer Prevention and Diagnosis

By utilizing the right tools, we can face cancer head-on with a full armor of protection. Throughout this book, we've spoken of a multitude of ways to help prevent cancer through things like diet, lifestyle, and supplementation. We also know we need to avoid certain toxins, pollutants, and harmful chemicals and foods. Each day we make decisions about what we'll put into our bodies and how we'll nourish ourselves. Part of nurturing and protecting ourselves also involves being proactive in other ways.

At our fingertips, we have a host of screening assessments readily available to us. Our doctors can help us order these tests; tests which may help us prevent cancer and save our lives. But we need to make the appointments. We need to notify healthcare providers when we're ill or experiencing odd symptoms. We need to make follow-up appointments and be accountable to ourselves.

We know that early detection of cancer IS life-saving. Finding cancer in its infancy greatly increases the chances for successful treatment. Recognizing possible warning signs of cancer and taking prompt action leads to early diagnosis. Not all cancers have warning signs, however, which is why screening is beneficial. Not everyone needs yearly or regular screening exams. If you are in the low-risk category, perhaps your screenings may be spaced out or even eliminated as time goes on. This is a conversation to have with your doctor. However, especially for individuals who've already had a primary cancer, routine screening is crucial and should be part of one's health maintenance regimen.

---

* Anticancer Action *

Get a yearly physical. Discuss with your doctor the tests and screenings that are recommended for you at this stage in your life.

Go to https://www.cancer.gov/about-cancer/screening/screening-tests for a complete list of cancer screenings.

Conclusion

Hopefully throughout this book, you've discovered some useful tools and strategies to help you create your healthiest body. You've learned about the healing effects of anti-angiogenic foods. You know that sugar and chemical-laden, processed foods cause ill health and just make you feel terrible. You've learned that even the best diet may be lacking in some nutrients, so carefully adding in certain supplements can boost your immune system and fill in the gaps. You understand that our world is filled with toxins, and even when we try to avoid them, they sneak into our systems. But, luckily you now also know of ways to detoxify your body. Most importantly, you also realize that taking care of YOU ... body, mind, and spirit ... is the greatest gift you can give yourself and your loved ones.

For those reading this who've already had a cancer diagnosis, it's important to know that cancer does NOT have to be a death sentence. You can implement healthy strategies outlined in this book starting tomorrow. You may be able to prevent a recurrence or a second cancer. Or, if you're currently undergoing treatment for cancer, you can incorporate things into your life that make you happy and bring you joy; things that fulfill your spirit and cause you to understand that you are so much more than your body.

Let's face it ... sometimes bad stuff happens to good people. Sometimes the healthiest, trimmest, fittest, happiest people get cancer. Sometimes, despite our best efforts, illness strikes. Whether our genes fail us or whether toxins unknowingly plague us, cancer can still be an unwelcome visitor in our bodies.

The reality is, we are mortal. But we need not be depressed or give into the notion that, "Life's a bitch, and then you die." Instead, let's think about how we can live life to its fullest. Let's make the most of our time here on this precious planet. When we take care of ourselves and our bodies, we can enjoy life so much more. We can have the energy to experience life in ways that bring us happiness. We can better love those around us when we love and nurture ourselves. We can glow from the inside out, and amazingly, that translates into our relationships. We gift others with our joy and show them that they, too, can feel wonderful.

Why not be the healthiest creature you can while you inhabit this world? We're put on this Earth for a short time. Life is not about biding our time and letting things just happen to us. Life is for pleasure and enjoyment. Life is for giving to others and fostering loving relationships. Being healthy and feeling good allows us the freedom to experience life to its fullest. Maybe you can't prevent all illness, but you sure can try. And even when our physical bodies begin to fail us, our spirits can soar. Nurturing ourselves includes not just nourishment from food but sustenance from prayer, meditation, laughter, and friendships. Let's agree to celebrate life and all that nature gives us. Let's care for ourselves, our environment, and each other. Let's enjoy our world and find joy in each day regardless of our circumstances.

You deserve to be happy and to be the best "you" you can be. That is your greatest gift to yourself and to the world.

"Self-care is not selfish or self-indulgent.
We cannot nurture others from a dry well.
We need to take care of our own needs first,
then we can give from our surplus, our abundance."
—Jennifer Louden

Shopping List

Stocking your refrigerator and pantry with nutrient-rich, anti-angiogenic foods is one of the greatest steps you can take towards wellness. Below is a list of some of foods to consider purchasing on your next shopping trip. Be sure to vary your produce from time to time, and try to eat seasonally. This ensures you're getting a variety of vitamins and minerals and that you're eating the freshest foods available. It's always best to try to buy organic when possible, but if that's not in the budget, traditional fruits and vegetables are still nutrient-dense and a good option. It's recommended to stick with organic, grass-fed, hormone-free meats and dairy products.

Vegetables	Fruits
Spinach	Red grapes
Kale	Strawberries
Bok choy	Blueberries
Swiss chard	Blackberries
Collard greens	Raspberries
Turnip greens	Cherries
Mustard greens	Oranges
Broccoli rabe	Lemons/Limes
Romaine	Grapefruit
Watercress	Apples
Arugula	Pineapple
Artichokes	Pumpkin

Vegetables (continued)
Parsley
Tomatoes
Garlic
Onions
Leeks
Shallots
Broccoli
Cauliflower
Radishes
Cabbage
Brussels sprouts
Edamame
Mushrooms
Bell peppers
Sweet potatoes
Carrots
Squash
Potatoes
Celery

Protein Sources
Tuna
Salmon
Herring
Trout
Mackerel
Sardines
Free-range eggs
Lamb

Fruits (continued)
Apricots
Cantaloupe
Honey dew
Watermelon
Pomegranate
Papaya
Guava
Kiwi
Plums
Prunes
Raisins
Cranberries (unsweetened)
Green bananas
Plantains

Nuts/Seeds
Walnuts
Pecans
Almonds
Brazil nuts
Flaxseed
Chia seeds
Hemp Seeds
Sunflower seeds
Sprouts
Almond butter
Sunflower seed butter
Organic peanut butter

Protein Sources (continued)

Grass-fed beef

Organ meats

Bone broths

Whey protein

Yogurt (plain, full fat)

Kefir

Chicken (with skin is fine if organic)

Pork (pastured)

Legumes

Kidney beans

Black beans

Split peas

Lentils

Peanuts

Grains

Gluten-free grains:

Quinoa

Wild rice

Brown rice

White rice

Oats

Buckwheat

Brown rice or quinoa pasta

Herbs / Spices

Turmeric

Nutmeg

Lavender

Cinnamon

Licorice

Allspice

Basil

Caraway

Cardamom

Clove

Cilantro

Cumin

Dill

Ginger

Rosemary

Saffron

Thyme

Himalayan sea salt

Fats / Oils

Olive oil

Coconut oil

Avocado oil

Avocado;

Grapeseed oil

Butter from grass-fed cows

Beverages

Green tea

Black tea

Dandelion tea

Licorice tea

Other herbal teas

Filtered water

Unsweetened coconut water

Coconut or almond milk
  (unsweetened)

Seltzer or sparkling water
  (unsweetened)

Red wine (in moderation)

Coffee

Fermented Foods

Sauerkraut

Pickles

Kimchi

Kombucha

Coconut kefir

Tempeh

Miso

Apple Cider Vinegar (organic,
  unfiltered)

Recipes with Anti-Angiogenic Ingredients

Cooking with a variety of vegetables, protein, and healthy fats is your best bet towards better health. If you're looking to reduce your cancer risk even further, concentrate on consuming anti-angiogenic foods (listed in Chapter 2). The following are recipes including some of those ingredients.

Sauteed Kale with Lemon

Ingredients:

1 bunch kale, washed, trimmed & cut into 2-inch pieces

1 tsp salt

2 T olive oil

1 T fresh lemon juice

1/4 tsp crushed red pepper (optional)

1/4 cup grated Parmesan cheese

1. Heat 1 inch of water in a large pot.

2. Add the kale and salt.

3. Cover & cook for about 5 minutes, stirring once, until crisp-tender.

4. Drain.

5. Return the kale to the pot.

6. Drizzle with olive oil.

7. Reheat.

8. Add the lemon juice, crushed red pepper, and parmesan.

9. Toss and serve.

**anti-angiogenic ingredients: kale, lemon, olive oil

**other anticancer ingredients: red pepper

Seared Tuna with Citrus Salsa

Ingredients:

2 tuna steaks (6-8 oz.)

2 oranges

1 red onion, chopped

1/2 cup cilantro, chopped

1 T olive oil

1 lime, juiced

salt

cayenne pepper (optional)

---

1. To make the salsa, section oranges, removing all peels and pith. Chop orange sections into 1/2-inch pieces.

2. Combine orange with onion, cilantro, olive oil, and lime juice. Toss together.

3. Season with salt and cayenne pepper to taste. Set aside.

4. Rub a cast iron grill pan with oil and heat.

5. Grill tuna, turning once, until desired degree of rareness is reached (2 to 5 minutes per side, depending on thickness).

6. Serve tuna topped with citrus salsa.

    **anti-angiogenic ingredients: tuna, orange, olive oil, lime

    **other anticancer ingredients: onion, cilantro, cayenne pepper

Pumpkin Soup

Ingredients:

6 cups chicken stock

1 1/2 tsp salt

4 cups pumpkin puree

1 tsp fresh parsley, chopped

1 cup onion, chopped

1/2 tsp fresh thyme, chopped

1 clove garlic, minced

1/2 cup heavy whipping cream

5 whole black peppercorns

1. Heat stock, salt, pumpkin, onion, thyme, garlic, and peppercorns.

2. Bring to a boil, reduce heat to low, and simmer for 30 minutes uncovered.

3. Puree the soup in small batches using a food processor or blender.

4. Return to pan and bring to boil again.

5. Reduce heat to low and simmer for another 30 minutes uncovered.

6. Stir in heavy cream.

7. Pour into soup bowls and garnish with fresh parsley.

   **anti-angiogenic ingredients: pumpkin, parsley, garlic

   **other anticancer ingredients: onion, thyme, black pepper

Roasted Artichokes

Ingredients:

4 large whole artichokes, top 1 inch and stems removed

1/4 cup fresh lemon juice

1/4 cup olive oil

4 cloves garlic, peeled and crushed

kosher salt

1. Preheat oven to 425 degrees F.
2. Place artichokes stem-side down in a bowl and drizzle with lemon juice
3. Slightly separate the artichoke leaves with your fingers.
4. Insert a knife blade into the center of each artichoke to create a garlic clove-size space.
5. Drizzle each artichoke with olive oil.
6. Press 1 clove of garlic into the center of each artichoke and season with salt.
7. Tightly wrap each artichoke with heavy-duty aluminum foil.
8. Place in baking dish and bake in the preheated oven until sizzling, about 1 hour 20 minutes.

**anti-angiogenic ingredients: artichokes, lemon, olive oil, garlic

Chili-Garlic Edamame

Ingredients:

1 pound frozen organic edamame in pods

1 T olive oil

1/4 tsp red pepper flakes

2 garlic cloves, minced

lime juice

salt

---

1. Cook edamame in boiling water until tender, about 5 minutes. Drain.

2. Heat olive oil, red pepper flakes, and garlic in a skillet over medium heat, 1-2 minutes.

3. Stir in the edamame.

4. Add lime juice and salt to taste.

    **anti-angiogenic ingredients: organic edamame, olive oil, garlic, lime

    **other anticancer ingredients: red pepper

Mushroom, Tomato, and Onion Saute

Ingredients:

2-4 T olive oil

2 onions, chopped

8 oz. mushrooms, quartered

4-5 medium tomatoes, chopped

salt and pepper, to taste

---

1. Preheat the pan over medium-low heat.
2. Add 2 T olive oil to pan.
3. Add the onions and brown slowly until tender and golden, about 10 minutes.
4. Add more oil if necessary, and add the mushrooms.
5. Cook an additional 10 minutes.
6. Add tomatoes and cook until soft, 10-15 minutes more.
7. Season with salt and pepper.
8. Serve atop wild rice, brown rice pasta, or grass-fed burgers.

   **anti-angiogenic ingredients: olive oil, mushrooms, tomatoes

   **other anticancer ingredients: onions, black pepper

Aloo Gobi
(Indian Style Cauliflower with Potatoes)

Ingredients:

1/4 cup olive oil

1 large onion chopped

1 bunch fresh cilantro; stalks removed, chopped, and reserved; leaves finely chopped

1 small green chili, chopped OR 1 tsp chili powder

1 large cauliflower, leaves removed and cut evenly into 8 segments

3 large potatoes, peeled and cubed

2 (8 oz.) cans diced tomatoes

1 tsp fresh ginger, peeled and grated

1 tsp fresh garlic, minced

1 tsp cumin seed

2 tsp turmeric

1 tsp salt

2 tsp garam masala spice blend

1. Heat oil in a large saucepan.

2. Add the onion and cumin seeds to the oil.

3. Stir together and cook until onions become golden and translucent.

4. Add cilantro stalks, turmeric, and salt.

5. Add chopped green chili to taste.

6. Stir tomatoes into onion mixture.

7. Add ginger and garlic. Mix thoroughly.

8. Add potatoes, stir, and cook for 10 minutes. (You may need to add some water to avoid sticking to the pan.)

9. Add the cauliflower and stir. Cook for an additional 20 minutes until potatoes are cooked.

10. Add garam masala and stir.

11. Sprinkle chopped cilantro leaves on top.

12. Turn off the heat, cover, and leave for as long as possible before serving.

13. Serve alone or with steamed rice or naan.

**anti-angiogenic ingredients: olive oil, tomatoes, garlic, turmeric

**other anticancer ingredients: onion, cilantro, ginger, cumin

Stir-Fried Bok Choy & Mushrooms

Ingredients:

1 lb bok choy

4 tsp olive oil

2 garlic cloves, minced

1 tsp fresh ginger, minced

5 oz. mushrooms, rinsed, de-stemmed

2 T rice wine or dry cooking sherry

1 T soy sauce (or coconut aminos to be gluten-free)

2 tsp sesame oil

1/8 tsp kosher salt

1/8 tsp black pepper

---

1. Trim away and chop bases of bok choy, and thinly slice leaves.

2. Heat oil in a large pan over medium heat.

3. Add garlic and ginger, stirring once.

4. Add mushrooms and stir-fry until they begin to brown, 1-2 minutes.

5. Add rice wine or sherry and cook 1 minute.

6. Add bok choy leaves and stalks. Toss, and cook until wilted, about 1 minute.

7. Add soy sauce or coconut aminos, sesame oil, salt and pepper.

8. Cook 1-2 minutes more, tossing frequently.

9. Serve with rice or rice noodles.

**anti-angiogenic ingredients: bok choy, olive oil, garlic, mushrooms

**other anticancer ingredients: ginger, black pepper

Crock-Pot Pineapple Chicken

Ingredients:

1 lb boneless, skinless chicken breasts

1 tsp paprika

1 tsp turmeric

1/2 tsp black pepper

20 oz. can pineapple chunks

2 T mustard

2 T tamari (wheat-free soy sauce)

1 clove garlic, minced

1 green pepper, chopped

red pepper flakes, to taste

1. Arrange chicken in bottom of crockpot.

2. Sprinkle with black pepper, turmeric, and paprika.

3. In a small bowl, combine pineapple, green pepper, mustard, tamari, and garlic.

4. Pour over chicken.

5. Sprinkle red pepper flakes over the chicken.

6. Cover and cook on Low 6-8 hours or on High 3-4 hours.

7. Serve with white or brown rice.

   **anti-angiogenic ingredients: pineapple, turmeric, garlic

   **other anticancer ingredients: black pepper, green pepper, red pepper flakes

Fruit & Kale Smoothie

Ingredients:

1 cup unsweetened vanilla almond milk

1/2 - 1 cup water (if needed)

1-2 cups kale, stems removed

1/2 cup frozen blueberries (or mixed berries)

1/4 cup frozen cherries

1/4 cup frozen pineapple

1 medium banana

1 T honey

2 T hydrolyzed collagen (if desired for added protein)

---

1. Put milk, kale, blueberries, cherries, pineapple, banana, honey, and collagen into a blender.

2. Blend on high until smooth and creamy.

3. If the consistency is too thick, add water and blend again.

4. Serve and drink immediately.

**anti-angiogenic ingredients: kale, blueberries, cherries, pineapple

**other anticancer ingredients: banana, hydrolyzed collagen

Crock-Pot Pork Chops with Apple, Onion, and Sweet Potato

Ingredients:

4 pork chops

2 onions, sliced into rings

2 sweet potatoes, peeled and sliced

2 Granny smith apples, peeled, cored, and sliced

3 T brown sugar

1 tsp cinnamon

1/2 tsp ground nutmeg

black pepper

salt

2 T chopped pecans

---

1. Place sweet potatoes in the bottom of the crockpot.

2. Layer the half the onions and apples on top.

3. Sprinkle with salt and pepper.

4. In a small bowl, combine the brown sugar, cinnamon, and nutmeg.

5. Sprinkle half of the brown sugar mixture on top.

6. Layer the pork chops next.

7. Sprinkle a pinch of salt and pepper over the chops.

8. Spread the other half of the onions and apples over the chops.

9. Sprinkle the rest of the brown sugar mixture over everything.

10. Cook on High for 4 hours or Low for 6-7 hours.

11. Serve with chopped pecans over each dish.

   **anti-angiogenic ingredients: apples, cinnamon, nutmeg

   **other anticancer ingredients: onions, sweet potatoes, pecans, black pepper

Wild Rice Cranberry Pecan Salad

Ingredients:

1 cup wild rice mix	1/4 cup sliced green onions
2 1/3 cups water (see rice instructions)	1 T lemon juice
	2 T olive oil
1/2 tsp salt	1/2 tsp sugar
1 tsp butter	1 tsp grated orange peel
1/2 cup dried unsweetened cranberries	salt
1/2 cup chopped pecans	pepper

1. Use the amount of water for the rice according to its instructions.

2. Bring rice, salt, butter, and water to a boil.

3. Reduce heat to low, cover and cook for 50 minutes. Do not stir or uncover.

4. Remove from stove and let sit covered for 10 minutes.

5. After 10 minutes, uncover, fluff with a fork, and let cool to almost room temperature.

6. In a medium bowl, mix the rice, cranberries, pecans, and green onions together.

7. In a separate jar, mix the lemon juice, olive oil, orange zest, sugar, and a pinch of salt and pepper. Shake.

8. Just prior to serving, mix the dressing in with the rice mixture.

9. May be served warm, chilled, or at room temperature.

**anti-angiogenic ingredients: lemon juice, olive oil, orange peel

**other anticancer ingredients: cranberries, pecans, onions, pepper

Wild Rice Meatballs

Ingredients:

1 1/4 lb grass-fed ground beef

1 organic egg, slightly beaten

1/2 cup onion, finely chopped

1 cup cooked wild rice

1 tsp salt

1 tsp garlic powder or minced garlic to taste

---

1. Preheat oven to 375 degrees F.

2. Combine ingredients and shape into 12 meatballs, about 2 inches in diameter.

3. Place meatballs on a baking sheet and bake for 30-40 minutes, until brown.

    **anti-angiogenic ingredients: garlic

    **other anticancer ingredients: grass-fed beef, organic egg, onion

Tuna-Stuffed Tomato Cups

Ingredients:

6 oz. light tuna, drained

2 hard boiled eggs, diced

1/2 cup celery, chopped

1 green onion, finely chopped

1 cup cook wild or brown rice

3 T mayonnaise

1 T fresh basil, chopped

1 T fresh dill, chopped

2 large tomatoes

---

1. Combine tuna, eggs, celery, onion, rice, and mayonnaise in a bowl.

2. Add basil and dill to taste.

3. Cut off the top and dig out the center of each tomato.

4. Divide tuna mixture evenly and spoon into each tomato cup.

   **anti-angiogenic ingredients: tuna, tomatoes

   **other anticancer ingredients: eggs (pasture-raised, organic), onion, celery, basil, dill

Crock-Pot Chicken and Wild Rice Soup

Ingredients:

1 medium onion, chopped

3 carrots, peeled and chopped

3 stalks of celery, chopped

2 cloves of garlic, finely chopped

1 cup uncooked wild rice, rinsed, and drained

2 bay leaves

1/2 tsp dried thyme

salt and black pepper, to taste

4 boneless, skinless chicken breasts

10 cups low-sodium chicken broth

1/4 cup chopped fresh parsley

1. In the crockpot, combine onion, carrots, celery, garlic, wild rice, bay leaves, thyme, salt and pepper.

2. Top with chicken breasts.

3. Add the chicken broth.

4. Place the lid on the crockpot, and cook on Low for 6 hours or High for 3 hours.

5. Carefully remove the chicken and shred using two forks.

6. Return chicken to the crockpot and stir.

7. Remove the bay leaves.

8. Add parsley and season with additional salt and pepper, to taste.

    **anti-angiogenic ingredients: garlic

    **other anticancer ingredients: onion, carrots, celery, thyme, parsley, black pepper

Walnut-Crusted Salmon

Ingredients:

1 1/2 cups walnuts	salt and pepper to taste
3 T dry breadcrumbs (preferably gluten-free)	6 (3 oz.) skin-on salmon fillets
3 T lemon rind, grated	Dijon mustard
1 1/2 T olive oil	2 T fresh lemon juice
3 T fresh dill, chopped	

---

1. Place walnuts in a food processor, and coarsely chop.

2. Add breadcrumbs, lemon rind, olive oil, and dill. Pulse until crumbly.

3. Season with salt and pepper, and set aside.

4. Arrange salmon fillets, skin side down, on foil-lined baking sheet.

5. Brush tops with mustard.

6. Spoon 1/3 cup of walnut mixture over each salmon fillet, and gently press the crumb mixture onto the surface of the fish.

7. Cover the baking sheet with plastic wrap and refrigerate for up to 2 hours.

8. Bake at 350 degrees F for 20 minutes, or until salmon flakes with a fork.

9. Before serving, sprinkle lemon juice over each piece of salmon.

   **anti-angiogenic ingredients: lemon, olive oil

   **other anticancer ingredients: walnuts, dill, pepper, salmon

Crock-Pot Chili

Ingredients:

2 lb grass-fed ground beef

1 large onion, chopped

2 garlic cloves, finely chopped

1 can (28 oz.) diced tomatoes, undrained

1 can (16 oz.) chili beans in sauce, undrained

1 can (15 oz.) tomato sauce

2 T chili powder

1 1/2 tsp ground cumin

1/2 tsp salt

1/2 tsp pepper

---

1. In a skillet, cook beef and onion until beef is brown, 8-10 minutes. Drain.

2. Mix beef and onion with the remaining ingredients in a crockpot.

3. Cover and cook on Low 6-8 hours.

   **anti-angiogenic ingredients: garlic, tomatoes, tomato sauce

   **other anticancer ingredients: grass-fed beef, onion, beans, chili powder, cumin, pepper

Broccoli Slaw

Ingredients:

1 large package broccoli cole slaw mix (or large head of cabbage shredded)

3 medium carrots, thinly sliced

3/4 mayonnaise or Greek yogurt

1 tsp mustard

1 tsp lemon juice

2 tsp apple cider vinegar

2 T honey

1/2 tsp salt

1/4 tsp pepper

1/2 tsp garlic powder

1/2 tsp basil

1/2 tsp parsley

1/2 tsp celery seed

---

1. Whisk mayo, mustard, lemon juice, ACV, honey, and spices until creamy.

2. Pour over broccoli slaw (or cabbage) and toss.

3. Refrigerate for at least 1 hour before serving.

**anti-angiogenic ingredients: lemon juice, parsley, garlic powder

**other anticancer ingredients: broccoli or cabbage, carrots, ACV, honey, pepper, basil, celery seed

Pumpkin Oat Bars

Ingredients:

1 1/2 cups quick-cooking, gluten-free oats

1/4 cup brown sugar

1 tsp baking powder

1 tsp cinnamon

1/2 tsp nutmeg

1/2 tsp pumpkin pie spice

1/2 tsp kosher salt

1/2 cup half-and-half (organic)

1 large organic egg

1 tsp vanilla extract

1 1/2 cups pumpkin puree

---

1. Preheat oven to 350 degrees F.

2. Grease an 8x8 inch baking pan.

3. In a bowl, stir together oats, brown sugar, baking powder, cinnamon, nutmeg, pumpkin pie spice, and salt.

4. Add half-and-half, egg, and vanilla extract to the mixture. Stir to combine.

5. Add the pumpkin puree, and mix thoroughly.

6. Pour pumpkin batter into prepared pan.

7. Bake 25-30 minutes, until a toothpick inserted in the middle comes out clean.

    **anti-angiogenic ingredients: cinnamon, nutmeg, pumpkin

    **other anticancer ingredients: oats, organic egg

Apple Cinnamon Overnight Oats

Ingredients:

1 1/2 cups gluten-free oats	1/4 tsp nutmeg
	1/2 tsp vanilla extract
1 1/2 cups unsweetened almond milk	1/2 cup water
2 T chia seeds	1 apple, cored and diced
1 T honey or maple syrup	1 cup walnuts, chopped
	1 T almond or peanut butter (optional)
1 tsp cinnamon	

---

1. Combine oats, almond milk, chia seeds, honey, cinnamon, nutmeg, vanilla, and water in a large glass container or jar. Stir to mix evenly.

2. Cover (or place lid on the jar), and refrigerate oat mixture overnight.

3. Remove from refrigerator. Using single serving mason jars, place a few spoonfuls of the oat mixture into the bottom of each jar.

4. Add a layer of diced apples, followed by a layer of walnuts.

5. Repeat layers until all ingredients are used up.

6. Store jars in the refrigerator up to 4 days.

7. When ready to eat, add an extra splash of almond milk, honey, and/or nut butter to taste.

8. May be eaten cold or warmed in the microwave for 30-60 seconds.

   **anti-angiogenic ingredients: apple, cinnamon, nutmeg

   **other anticancer ingredients: oats, chia seeds, honey, walnuts, nut butter

Black Bean Brownies

Ingredients:

1/4 cup coconut oil

1/4 cup dark chocolate chips

1/4 cup cocoa powder

1/4 cup unsweetened apple sauce

3 organic eggs

1 can black beans, drained and rinsed

1/2 tsp vanilla extract

1/4 tsp salt

1/4 cup chopped nuts (optional)

---

1. Preheat oven to 350 degrees F.

2. Grease an 8x8 inch baking dish.

3. Melt the coconut oil and chocolate chips together in the microwave or double boiler.

4. Combine the melted coconut oil and chocolate chips with the remaining ingredients in a blender.

5. Puree until smooth.

6. Stir in the optional chopped nuts if desired.

7. Pour into prepared baking dish, and bake for 35-40 minutes or until set.

   **anti-angiogenic ingredients: dark chocolate, cocoa powder, unsweetened apple sauce

   **other anticancer ingredients: coconut oil, organic eggs, black beans, nuts

No-Bake Chocolate Coconut Cookies

Ingredients:

2 1/2 cups gluten-free rolled oats	1/2 cup coconut oil
	1 cup almond butter
1 cup unsweetened shredded coconut flakes	2 tsp vanilla extract
2-3 T dark chocolate chips	6 T cocoa powder
	coconut sugar
2/3 cup honey	Himalayan sea salt

1. Line 2 baking sheets with parchment paper and set aside.

2. In a large bowl, mix the oats and coconut flakes together and set aside.

3. In a medium pot over medium heat, combine honey, coconut oil, almond butter, and cocoa powder. Stir continuously until the mixture is melted and mixed evenly.

4. Remove from heat and add in the oats/coconut mixture and the chocolate chips, and stir well.

5. Add the vanilla extract and continue stirring until mixture becomes thick.

6. Drop heaping tablespoons onto the prepared baking sheets.

7. Lightly sprinkle a bit of coconut sugar and Himalayan sea salt on top of each cookie.

8. Place the baking sheets into the freezer for about 20 minutes or until ready to serve.

9. Allow the cookies to thaw for about 5 minutes before serving.

10. Store leftover cookies in a sealed container in the freezer.

    **anti-angiogenic ingredients: dark chocolate, cocoa powder

    **other anticancer ingredients: oats, coconut, honey, coconut oil, almond butter

Bibliography

"10 Natural Cancer Treatments Revealed." *Dr. Axe*, Accessed 23 May 2017, https://draxe.com/10-natural-cancer-treatments-hidden-cures/.

Laliberte, Richard. "20 Ways to Never Get Cancer." *Prevention*, 16 Nov. 2011, http://www.prevention.com/health/health-concerns/everyday-cancer-prevention-tips.

"New Natural Way to Starve Cancer and Obesity." *Mercola*, 8 June 2010, http://articles.mercola.com/sites/articles/archive/2010/06/08/dramatically-effective-new-natural-way-to-starve-cancer-and-obesity.aspx.

Park, Alice. "The Curious Link Between Allergies and Cancer." *Healthland*, TIME, 12 July 2011, http://healthland.time.com/2011/07/12/the-curious-link-between-allergies-and-cancer/.

"Why Are There So Many Food Allergies Now?" *Mercola*, 14 June 2011, http://articles.mercola.com/sites/articles/archive/2011/06/14/why-are-there-so-many-food-allergies-now.aspx.

Tate, Nick. "Allergies Raise Cancer Risk: Study." *Newsmax Health*, 30 April 2015, http://www.newsmax.com/Health/Health-News/allergy-inflammation-cancer/2015/04/30/id/641794/.

"Cancer Statistics." *National Cancer Institute*. NIH, 22 March 2017, https://www.cancer.gov/about-cancer/understanding/statistics.

"Common Cancer Myths and Misconceptions." *National Cancer Institute*. NIH, 3 Feb. 2014, https://www.cancer.gov/about-cancer/causes-prevention/risk/myths.

"Cancer Causes." *Mayo Clinic*. 23 May 2015, http://www.mayoclinic.org/diseases-conditions/cancer/basics/causes/con-20032378.

Ravindran, Jayaraj, et al. "Curcumin and Cancer Cells: How Many Ways Can Curry Kill Cancer Cells Selectively?" *AAPS Journal*, 2009 Sep; 11(3): 495–510. *PubMed* PMID: PMC2758121.

Kaefer, Christine M. and John A. Milner. "Herbs and Spices in Cancer Prevention and Treatment." *Herbal Medicine: Biomolecular and Clinical Aspects*. 2011; Pub Med Bookshelf ID: NBK92774PMID: 22593940.

Nair, Suresh. "3 Anti-Cancer Health Benefits of Green Tea." *The Truth About Cancer*, Accessed 24 May 2017, https://thetruthaboutcancer.com/three-anti-cancer-health-benefits-of-green-tea/.

Weller, Chris. "Olive Oil Compound Kills Cancer Cells in Less Than an Hour: All-Powerful Oleancanthal." *Medical Daily*, 20 Feb. 2015, http://www.medicaldaily.com/olive-oil-compound-kills-cancer-cells-less-hour-all-powerful-oleocanthal-322904.

Wen, Wei, et al. "Grape Seed Extract (GSE) Inhibits Angiogenesis Via Suppressing VEGFR Signaling Pathway." *Cancer Prev Res (Phila)*. 2008 Dec; 1(7): 554-561. PubMed PMCID: PMC2802543.

Kleczewski, Krista and Claire Karisson. "Can a Handful of Nuts a Day Keep Cancer Away?" *Stop Cancer Fund*, 2015, http://www.stopcancerfund.org/p-breast-cancer/can-a-handful-of-nuts-a-day-keep-cancer-away/.

Oxford University Press (OUP). "Nuts and peanuts -- but not peanut butter -- linked to lower mortality rates, study finds." *ScienceDaily*. ScienceDaily, 10 June 2015. <www.sciencedaily.com/releases/2015/06/150610190920.htm>.

Guasch-Ferré, Marta, et al. "Frequency of nut consumption and mortality risk in the PREDIMED nutrition intervention trial." 2013 *BMC Med*; 11: 164. doi: 10.1186/1741-7015-11-164.

Toner, CD., "Communicating clinical research to reduce cancer risk through diet: Walnuts as a case example." 2014, July 28. *Nutr Res Pract*. 8(4): 347–351. doi: 10.4162/nrp.2014.8.4.347.

Greger, Michael M.D. "Which Nut Fights Cancer Better?" *Nutrition Facts*, 18 July 2014, https://nutritionfacts.org/video/which-nut-fights-cancer-better/.

Soriano-Hernandez AD, et al. "The Protective Effect of Peanut, Walnut, and Almond Consumption on the Development of Breast Cancer." *Gynecologic and Obstetric Investigation*. 2015 Jul 10; PubMed PMID: 26183374 DOI: 10.1159/000369997.

Ip C, Lisk DJ. "Bioactivity of Selenium from Brazil Nut for Cancer Prevention and Selenoenzyme Maintenance." Nutrition and Cancer. 1994;21(3):203-12; PMID: 8072875 DOI: 10.1080/01635589409514319.

"7 Benefits of Eating Hemp Seeds You Won't Believe." *Dr. Axe*, Accessed 24 May 2017, https://draxe.com/7-hemp-seed-benefits-nutrition-profile/.

"AICR's Foods That Fight Cancer." American Institute for Cancer Research, Accessed 24 May 2017, http://www.aicr.org/foods-that-fight-cancer/.

Dhar A, Mehta S, Dhar G, et al. "Crocetin inhibits pancreatic cancer cell proliferation and tumor progression in a xenograft mouse model." *Mol Cancer Ther*. 2009 Feb;8(2):315-23.

Zhang, Li and Handong Wang. "Multiple Mechanisms of Anti-cancer Effects Exerted by Astaxanthin." *Marine Drugs*. 2015 Jul; 13(7): 4310–4330; PMCID: PMC4515619; doi: 10.3390/md13074310.

Kresser, Chris. "Red Meat and Cancer—Again! Will It Ever Stop?" *Chris Kresser*, 29 October 2015, https://chriskresser.com/red-meat-cancer-again-will-it-ever-stop/.

Roe, Matthew. "The Cancer Fighting Benefits of Whey Protein." *Natural Health 365*, 24 March 2014, http://www.naturalhealth365.com/0943_whey_protein.html/.

Konarikova, Katarina, et al. "Anticancer Effect of Black Tea Extract in Human Cancer Cell Lines." *SpringerPlus*, 2015 Mar 14; PMCID: PMC4374083; doi: 10.1186/s40064-015-0871-4.

"Five Reasons to Skip Bottled Water." *EWG*, 22 Sep. 2013, http://www.ewg.org/research/ewgs-water-week.

Group, Dr. Edward. "12 Toxins in Your Drinking Water." *Global Healing Center*, 3 May 2016, http://www.globalhealingcenter.com/natural-health/12-toxins-in-your-drinking-water/.

"Chemicals in Meat Cooked at High Temperatures and Cancer Risk." *National Cancer Institute*, NIH, 19 October 2015, https://www.cancer.gov/about-cancer/causes-prevention/risk/diet/cooked-meats-fact-sheet.

Ren, Jian-Song, et al. "Pickled Food and Risk of Gastric Cancer—A Systematic Review and Meta-analysis of English and Chinese Literature." *Cancer Epidemiology, Biomarkers, & Prevention*; AACR Publications, June 2012, http://cebp.aacrjournals.org/content/21/6/905.

Fritz, W and Soos, K. "Smoked Food and Cancer." *Bibl Nutr Dieta*. 1980;(29):57-64; PMID: 7447916.

Genkinger, Jeanine, and Koushik, Anita. "Meat Consumption and Cancer Risk." *PLOS Med*. 2007 Dec; PMCID: PMC2121650; doi: 10.1371/journal.pmed.0040345.

Walton, Alice. "Why High Protein Diets May be Linked to Cancer Risk." *Forbes*, 4 Mar 2014, https://www.forbes.com/sites/alicegwalton/2014/03/04/the-protein-puzzle-meat-and-dairy-may-significantly-increase-cancer-risk/#24790dc558b7.

Richman, EL et al. "Choline Intake and Risk of Lethal Prostate Cancer: Incidence and Survival." *Am J Clin Nutr.* 2012 Oct;96(4):855-63; PMID: 22952174 PMCID: PMC3441112 DOI: 10.3945/ajcn.112.039784.

Rafie N, et al. "Kefir and Cancer: A Systematic Review of Literatures." *Arch Iran Med.* 2015 Dec;18(12):852-7. doi: 0151812/AIM.0011; PMID: 26621019.

Siri-Tarino, Patty et al. "Meta-analysis of Prospective Cohort Studies Evaluating the Association of Saturated Fat with Cardiovascular Disease." *The American Journal of Clinical Nutrition,* January 13, 2010, doi: 10.3945/ ajcn.2009.2772.

Lundell, Dwight. "World Renown Heart Surgeon Speaks Out On What Really Causes Heart Disease." *Prevent Disease,* 1 March 2012, http://preventdisease.com/news/12/030112_World-Renown-Heart-Surgeon-Speaks-Out-On-What-Really-Causes-Heart-Disease.shtml.

Boyd, DB. "Insulin and Cancer." *Integr Cancer Ther.* 2003 Dec;2(4):315-29; PMID: 14713323 DOI: 10.1177/1534735403259152.

Anderson L.A. et al. "Malignancy and mortality in a population-based cohort of patients with coeliac disease or 'gluten sensitivity'". *World Journal of Gastroenterology.* 2007 Jan 7;13(1):146-51.

Hoggan R. "Considering wheat, rye, and barley proteins as aids to carcinogens." *Medical Hypotheses.* 1997 Sep;49(3):285-8.

Ettinger, Jill. "Everything You Absolutely Need to Know About GMOs." *Organic Authority,* 20 Feb. 2012, https://www.organicauthority.com/foodie-buzz/what-are-gmos-genetically-modified-crops-foods.html.

Gao, Hui, et al. "Bisphenol A and Hormone-Associated Cancers: Current Progress and Perspectives." *Medicine (Baltimore).* 2015 Jan; 94(1): e211; PMCID: PMC4602822.

"Alcohol and Cancer Risk." *National Cancer Institute*, NIH, 24 June 2013, https://www.cancer.gov/about-cancer/causes-prevention/risk/alcohol/alcohol-fact-sheet.

Vioque, Jesus, et al. "Esophageal Cancer risk by type of alcohol drinking and smoking: a case-control study in Spain." *BMC Cancer*. 2008 Aug 1, doi: 10.1186/1471-2407-8-221; PMCID: PMC2529333.

David, Yair Bar, et al. "Water Intake and Cancer Prevention." *Journal of Clinical Oncology*, Jan. 2014, DOI: 10.1200/JCO.2004.99.245; 383-385; PMID: 14722055.

Morris, RD. "Drinking Water and Cancer." *Environmental Health Perspectives*. 1995 Nov; 103(Suppl 8): 225–23; PMCID: PMC1518976.

Block, G. "Vitamin C and Cancer Prevention: The Epidemiologic Evidence." *Am J Clin Nutr*. 1991 Jan;53(1 Suppl):270S-282S; PMID: 1985398.

Prasad, AS, et al. "Zinc in Cancer Prevention." *Nutr Cancer*. 2009;61(6):879-87. doi: 10.1080/01635580903285122; PMID: 20155630.

Donaldson, Michael S. "Nutrition and Cancer: A Review of the Evidence for An Anti-cancer Diet." *Nutr J*. 2004 Oct 20. doi: 10.1186/1475-2891-3-19; PMCID: PMC526387.

"How Selenium Helps Protect Against Cancer." *The Physicians Committee for Responsible Medicine*, Accessed 25 May 2017, https://www.pcrm.org/health/cancer-resources/diet-cancer/nutrition/how-selenium-helps-protect-against-cancer.

Ehrlich, Steven. "Omega-3 Fatty Acids." *University of Maryland Medical Center*, 5 Aug. 2015, http://www.umm.edu/health/medical/altmed/supplement/omega3-fatty-acids.

Jayathilake, A., et al. "Krill Oil Extract Suppresses Cell Growth and Induces Apoptosis of Human Colorectal Cancer Cells." *BMC Complement Altern Med*. 2016 Aug 30; 16(1): 328 doi: 10.1186/s12906-016-1311-x PMCID: PMC5004275.

Ding, Jin-Feng, et al. "Study on Effect of Jellyfish Collagen Hydrolysate on Anti-fatigue and Anti-oxidation." *Science Direct*, 4 Jan. 2011, http://www.sciencedirect.com/science/article/pii/S0268005X10 002961.

Kojima, T., et al. "Effect of Gelatins on Human Cancer Cells in Vitro." *Cancer Biother Radiopharm*. 2003 Apr;18(2):147-55; PMID: 12804040 DOI: 10.1089/108497803765036319.

"Can Turmeric Prevent or Treat Breast Cancer?" *Cancer Research UK*, 6 Aug. 2015, http://www.cancerresearchuk.org/about-cancer/cancers-in-general/cancer-questions/can-turmeric-prevent-bowel-cancer.

Kumar, M., et al. "Cancer-Preventing Attributes of Probiotics: An Update." *Int J Food Sci Nutr*. 2010 Aug;61(5):473-96. doi: 10.3109/09637480903455971; PMID: 20187714.

"Probiotics Benefits, Foods and Supplements." *Dr. Axe*, Accessed 25 May 2017, https://draxe.com/probiotics-benefits-foods-supplements/.

"Diindolylmethane." *Memorial Sloan Kettering Cancer Center*, 18 Feb. 2016, https://www.mskcc.org/cancer-care/integrative-medicine/herbs/diindolylmethane.

Kaur, Majinder, et al. "Anticancer and Cancer Chemopreventive Potential of Grape Seed Extract and Other Grape-Based Products." *Journal of Nutrition*. 2009 Sep; 139(9): 1806S–1812S; doi: 10.3945/jn.109.106864; PMCID: PMC2728696.

Turner, Ashley. "Essential Oils for Cancer Support." *MindBodyGreen*, 18 Apr 2013, https://www.mindbodygreen.com/0-8823/essential-oils-for-cancer-support.html.

Mills, EJ., et al. "Low-dose Aspirin and Cancer Mortality: a Meta-analysis of Randomized Trials." *Am J Med*. 2012 Jun;125(6):560-7. doi: 10.1016/j.amjmed.2012.01.017. Epub 2012 Apr 17.

Verkerk, Robert. "Does Folic Acid Protect From - or Cause-Cancer?" *ANH International*, 12 Feb. 2014, http://anhinternational.org/2014/02/12/anh-intl-feature-does-folic-acid-protect-from-or-cause-cancer/.

Challem, Jack. "Natural vs. Synthetic Vitamin E." *Nutrition Science News*, Accessed 25 May 2017, http://www.chiro.org/nutrition/FULL/Natural_vs_Synthetic_Vitamin_E.shtml.

"Is There a Link Between Birth Control Pills and Higher Breast Cancer Risk?" *BreastCancer.org*, 4 Aug. 2014, http://www.breastcancer.org/research-news/study-questions-birth-control-and-risk.

"Women's Health Initiative." *Wikipedia*, Accessed 25 May 2017, https://en.wikipedia.org/wiki/Women's_Health_Initiative.

Ogilvy-Stuart, AL. and H. Gleeson. "Cancer Risk Following Growth Hormone Use in Childhood: implications for current practice." *Drug Safety*. 2004;27(6):369-82; PMID: 15144231.

Sorensen, Henrik, et al. "Skin Cancers and Non-Hodgkin Lymphoma Among Users of Systemic Glucocorticoids: A Population-Based Cohort Study." *J Natl Cancer Inst* (2004) 96 (9): 709-711; DOI: https://doi.org/10.1093/jnci/djh118.

Velicer, Christine, et al. "Antibiotic Use in Relation to the Risk of Breast Cancer." *The JAMA Network*, 18 Feb. 2004; 291(7):827-835. doi:10.1001/jama.291.7.827.

"Antibiotics and Cancer." *PBS NewsHour*, PBS WQED, 17 Feb. 2004, http://www.pbs.org/newshour/bb/health-jan-june04-cancer_02-17/.

Condrea-Rado, Anna. "Can Dry Cleaning Give You Cancer? The Hidden Hazards of Delicates." *The Guardian*, 18 Nov. 2016, https://www.theguardian.com/lifeandstyle/2016/nov/18/dry-cleaning-toxic-process-carcinogen-cancer.

Choi, Anna, et al. "Developmental Fluoride Neurotoxicity: A Systematic Review and Meta-Analysis." *Environ Health Prospect.* 2012 Oct; 120(10): 1362–1368; doi: 10.1289/ehp.1104912; PMCID: PMC3491930.

Peckham, Steven and Niyi Awofeso. "Water Fluoridation: A Critical Review of the Physiological Effects of Ingested Fluoride as a Public Health Intervention." *Scientific World Journal.* 2014: 293019; 2014 Feb 26. doi: 10.1155/2014/293019; PMCID: PMC3956646.

Chandna, Shalu and Manish Bathla. "Oral Manifestations of Thyroid Disorders and Its Management." *Indian J Endocrinol Metab.* 2011 Jul; 15(Suppl2): S113–S116; doi: 10.4103/2230-8210.83343; PMCID: PMC3169868.

Bassin, EB et al. "Age-specific fluoride exposure in drinking water and osteosarcoma (United States)." *Cancer Causes Control.* 2006 May;17(4):421-8. PMID: 16596294 DOI: 10.1007/s10552-005-0500-6.

"Skip the Non-Stick to Avoid the Dangers of Teflon." *EWG*, Accessed 25 May 2017, http://www.ewg.org/research/healthy-home-tips/tip-6-skip-non-stick-avoid-dangers-teflon.

Sholl, Jessie. "8 Hidden Toxins: What's Lurking in Your Cleaning Products?" *Experience Life*, Oct. 2011, https://experiencelife.com/article/8-hidden-toxins-whats-lurking-in-your-cleaning-products/.

"Cell Phones and Cancer Risk." *National Cancer Institute,* NIH, 27 May 2016, https://www.cancer.gov/about-cancer/causes-prevention/risk/radiation/cell-phones-fact-sheet.

"5 Ways to Reduce Cell Phone Radiation Exposure." *Empowered Sustenance*, 14 June 2014, http://empoweredsustenance.com/cell-phone-radiation/.

Storrs, Carina. "How Much Do CT Scans Increase the Risk of Cancer?" *Scientific American*, 1 Jul. 2013, https://www.scientificamerican.com/article/how-much-ct-scans-increase-risk-cancer/.

"Frequently Asked Questions about HPV Vaccine Safety." *CDC*, 23 Jan. 2017, https://www.cdc.gov/vaccinesafety/vaccines/hpv/hpv-safety-faqs.html#A2.

"Pre-exposure Prophylaxis (PrEP) HIV Risk and Prevention." CDC, 17 Apr. 2017, https://www.cdc.gov/hiv/risk/prep/.

McDermott, Annette. "Natural Treatment for H. pylori: What Works?" *Healthline*, 10 Aug. 2016, http://www.healthline.com/health/digestive-health/h-pylori-natural-treatment#Naturaltreatments2.

Giovannucci, Edward, et al. "Diabetes and Cancer." *Diabetes Care*. 2010 Jul; 33(7): 1674–1685; doi: 10.2337/dc10-0666; PMCID: PMC2890380.

Frans, Alexis and Jill Slansky. "Multiple Associations Between a Broad Spectrum of Autoimmune Diseases, Chronic Inflammatory Diseases and Cancer." *Anticancer Res.* 2012 Apr; 32(4): 1119–1136.PMCID: PMC3349285, NIHMSID: NIHMS372423.

"Allergies and Cancer: A Connection?" *Achoo Allergy*, Accessed 25 May 2017, https://www.achooallergy.com/learning/allergy-cancer-is-there-a-connection/.

"More Evidence of Exercise for Cancer Prevention." *American Institute for Cancer Research*, 18 May 2016, http://www.aicr.org/cancer-research-update/2016/05_18/cru-More-Evidence-of-Exercise-for-Cancer-Prevention.html.

Gibala, Martin, et al. "Short-term sprint interval *versus* traditional endurance training: similar initial adaptations in human skeletal muscle and exercise performance." *Journal of Physiology*, The Physiological Society, 6 Sep. 2006, 575: 901–911. doi:10.1113/jphysiol.2006.112094.

"Sedentary Behavior Increases the Risk of Certain Cancers." *J Natl Cancer Inst* (2014); 106 (7): dju206; DOI: https://doi.org/10.1093/jnci/dju206.

Taylor, Shelley et al. "Biobehavioral Responses to Stress in Females: Tend-and-Befriend, Not Fight-or-Flight." *Psychological Review* 2000, Vol.107, No. 3, 411-429; https://scholar.harvard.edu/marianabockarova/files/tend-and-befriend.pdf.

Moran, Victoria. "Reduced Stress — The Health Benefits of Friendship." *Cleveland Clinic Wellness*, 29 June 2010, http://www.clevelandclinicwellness.com/mind/stressless/Pages/TheHealthBenefitsofFriendship.aspx.

Holt-Lunstad, Julianna et al. "Social Relationships and Mortality Risk: A Meta-analytic Review." *PLOS Medicine*, 27 July 2010, doi.org/10.1371/journal.pmed.1000316.

"Epsom Salt Uses and Benefits." *Salt Works*, Accessed 25 May 2017, https://www.seasalt.com/bath/epsom-salt-uses-and-benefits.

"Frequent religious service attendance linked with decreased mortality risk among women." *Harvard T.H.Chan School of Public Health*, 16 May 2016, https://www.hsph.harvard.edu/news/press-releases/religious-service-attendance-womens-mortality-risk/.

"Why Is Sleep Important?" *National Heart, Lung, and Blood Institute*, NIH, 22 Feb. 2012, https://www.nhlbi.nih.gov/health/health-topics/topics/sdd/why.

"Researchers are Studying the Link Between Sleep and Cancer." *Cancer Treatment Centers of America*, Accessed 25 May 2017, http://www.cancercenter.com/community/newsletter/article/researchers-are-studying-the-link-between-sleep-and-cancer/.

Exelmans, Liese and Jan Van den Bulck. "Bedtime Mobile Phone Use and Sleep in Adults." *Social Science and Medicine*, Volume 148, January 2016, Pages 93–101, Science Direct, http://www.sciencedirect.com/science/article/pii/S027795361530245 8.

Cordeiro, Brittany. "Breastfeeding Lowers Your Breast Cancer Risk." *University of Texas MD Anderson Cancer Center*, Oct 2014, https://www.mdanderson.org/publications/focused-on-health/october-2014/breastfeeding-breast-cancer-prevention.html.

Oaklander, Mandy. "Breastfeeding Linked to a Lower Risk of Cancer in Kids." *TIME Health*, 1 Jun 2015, http://time.com/3901565/breastfeeding-childhood-cancer-leukemia/.

"Obesity and Cancer." *National Cancer Institute*, NIH, 17 January 2017, https://www.cancer.gov/about-cancer/causes-prevention/risk/obesity/obesity-fact-sheet#q4.

Leitzmann, Michael et al. "Ejaculation Frequency and Subsequent Risk of Prostate Cancer." *JAMA*, 2004;291(13):1578-1586. doi:10.1001/jama.291.13.1578.

Magee, Anna. "Sex is Good For You: For Fighting Cancer to the Common Cold It's Just What the Doctor Ordered (And Men Benefit Most!)" *Daily Mail*, 10 Feb 2009, http://www.dailymail.co.uk/health/article-1140388/Sex-good-For-fighting-cancer-common-cold-just-doctor-ordered-men-benefit-most.html.

Nichols, Helen. "How to Detox Your Body: 35 Natural Strategies." *Well-Being Secrets*, Accessed 26 May 2017, http://www.well-beingsecrets.com/detox-of-your-body-35-natural-ways/.

Teodorczyk-Injeyan, JA et al. "Spinal Manipulative Therapy Reduces Inflammatory Cytokines but Not Substance P Production in Normal Subjects." *J Manipulative Physiol Ther.* 2006 Jan;29(1):14-21.PMID: 16396725 DOI: 10.1016/j.jmpt.2005.10.002.

Prinster, Tari. "Five Ways That Yoga Helps Prevent Cancer." *Kripalu Center For Yoga and Health*, Accessed 26 May 2017, https://kripalu.org/resources/five-ways-yoga-helps-prevent-cancer.

Jamieson, Alex. "Why Water is the Key to Detoxifying Your Body." *VegKitchen*, Accessed 26 May 2017, http://www.vegkitchen.com/nutrition/water-detoxifying/.

Klement, Rainer et al. "Is there a role for carbohydrate restriction in the treatment and prevention of cancer?" *Nutrition and Metabolism (London).* 2011 Oct 26. doi: 10.1186/1743-7075-8-75; PMCID: PMC3267662.

"Understanding Your Risk of Developing Secondary Cancers." *National Comprehensive Cancer Network*, 2017, https://www.nccn.org/patients/resources/life_after_cancer/understanding.aspx.

"Accuracy of Mammograms." *Susan G. Komen*, 22 July 2016, http://ww5.komen.org/BreastCancer/AccuracyofMammograms.html.

"Mammogram Basics." *American Cancer Society*, Accessed 26 May 2017, https://www.cancer.org/cancer/breast-cancer/screening-tests-and-early-detection/mammograms/mammogram-basics.html.

"Breast Cancer Statistics." *Cancer.Net*. Apr 2017, http://www.cancer.net/cancer-types/breast-cancer/statistics.

"What Is Breast Thermography?" *American College of Clinical Thermology*, Accessed 27 May 2017, http://www.thermologyonline.org/Breast/breast_thermography_what.htm.

"Breast Cancer (BRCA) Gene Test." *WebMD*, Accessed 27 May 2017, http://www.webmd.com/breast-cancer/breast-cancer-brca-gene-test#4.

"What Are the Risk Factors For Ovarian Cancer?" *American Cancer Society*, 4 Feb 2016, https://www.cancer.org/cancer/ovarian-cancer/causes-risks-prevention/risk-factors.html.

"Loop Electrocautery Excision Procedure (LEEP) and Cone Biopsy." *UW Medicine*, Accessed 27 May 2016, http://www.uwmedicine.org/health-library/Pages/loop-electrocautery-excision-procedure-leep-and-cone-biopsy.aspx.

"HPV and HPV Testing." *American Cancer Society*, 12 April 2016, https://www.cancer.org/cancer/cancer-causes/infectious-agents/hpv/hpv-and-hpv-testing.html.

"Skin Cancer Facts and Statistics." *Skin Cancer Foundation*, 2 Feb 2017, http://www.skincancer.org/skin-cancer-information/skin-cancer-facts#melanoma.

"Lung Cancer Risk Factors." *American Cancer Society*, 22 Feb 2016, https://www.cancer.org/cancer/lung-cancer/prevention-and-early-detection/risk-factors.html.

"Signs and Symptoms of Liver Cancer." *American Cancer Society*, 28 Apr 2016, https://www.cancer.org/cancer/liver-cancer/detection-diagnosis-staging/signs-symptoms.html.

"Secondary Malignancies." *UNM Comprehensive Cancer Center*, Accessed 28 May 2017, http://cancer.unm.edu/cancer/cancer-info/cancer-treatment/side-effects-of-cancer-treatment/long-term-side-effects/secondary-malignancies/.

"Second Cancers." *Livestrong*, Accessed 28 May 2017, https://www.livestrong.org/we-can-help/healthy-living-after-treatment/second-cancers.

Jockers, David. "The Healing Benefits of Hyperbaric Oxygen Therapy." *The Truth About Cancer*, Accessed 28 May 2017, https://thetruthaboutcancer.com/hyperbaric-oxygen-therapy/.

"Do You Have a Wheat Belly? Interview with Dr. William Davis." *Wellness Mama*, 24 March 2017, https://wellnessmama.com/3486/dr-william-davis-wheat-belly/.

Runyon, Joel. "Are Artificial Sweeteners Paleo?" *Ultimate Paleo Guide*, 6 October 2013, https://ultimatepaleoguide.com/are-artificial-sweeteners-paleo/.

"The 5 Worst Artificial Sweeteners." *Dr. Axe*, Accessed 10 July 2017, https://draxe.com/artificial-sweeteners/.

"Effects of GMOs on Children." *Earthbeam Natural Foods*, 2016, http://earthbeamfoods.blogspot.com/2013/03/gmo-series-5-effects-of-gmos-on-children.html.

Some recipes have been adapted from the following websites: foodnetwork.com, allrecipes.com, food.com, myrecipes.com, weightandwellness.com, twopeasandtheirpod.com, walnuts.org, bettycrocker.com, wellnessmama.com, thatcleanlife.com, draxe.com.

About the Author

KIM MARAVICH'S background as an RN fostered her passion for nutrition and preventative healthcare. She also has an MA in Teaching and enjoys educating and encouraging others to optimize their health. She has published articles about varying health issues, vitamin and mineral supplementation, superfoods, and children's health.

Kim lives just outside of Pittsburgh, PA, with her husband and two young boys. You can follow her at www.facebook.com/kimmaravichhealthwriter/ and at her website kimmaravich.com. Some of her articles can also be found at kimmaravich.hubpages.com.

Made in the USA
San Bernardino, CA
22 May 2018